NEVER
Act Your Age

Play the Happy Childlike Role
Well at Every Age

Keep Laughing for the
Health of it!

Dale L. Anderson, M.D.
with Arden Moore

[signature: Dale Anderson M.D.]

Beaver's P
Edina,

ISBN 1-931646-38-4

Library of Congress Catalog Number: 2002103799

Printed in the United States of America

First Printing: April 2002

06 05 04 03 02   6 5 4 3 2 1

Beaver's Pond Press, Inc.   5125 Danen's Drive
Edina, MN 55439-1465
(952) 829-8818
www.beaverspondpress.com

to order, visit midwestbookhouse.com or call 1-877-430-0044. Quantity discounts available.

DEDICATION

This book celebrates thousands of role model patient-friends who had their act together. Over the years, they have been my SHE-roes and HE-roes—in living and in dying.

They laughed with me, cried with me, and always shared the conviction that life is a gift. A happy gift. A miracle gift. A gift that should be enjoyed, cherished, and lived with passion.

This book is gratefully dedicated to patients who doctored the doctor.

D.L.A.

IMPORTANT NOTE TO READERS

This book, *Never Act Your Age*, is intended for general information only. It cannot substitute for personalized medical care or prescribed treatment. I recommend you seek the guidance of a licensed physician or healthcare professional before making any changes or additions to treatment approaches. You are advised to have your personal health care provider evaluate the suggestions offered in this book prior to their use.

If you have, or suspect a medical problem, I urge you to pursue competent medical health care. NOW!

D.L.A.
St. Paul, Minnesota

THE CAST OF "CHARACTERS"

DALE ANDERSON, M.D.—has practiced for over 40 years as a family physician, board-certified surgeon, and board-certified emergency physician. He currently practices as an urgent care doctor. He is also certified as a Diplomate of the American Board of Holistic Medicine. As a keynote/seminar speaker, this Minnesota native prescribes METHOD acting techniques to more than 100 major audiences around the world each year. His one man "medicine show" dispenses healthy, happy INNER-tainment at its best. The author of four books, he can be reached through his web site: www.acthappy.com

ARDEN MOORE—An award-winning writer who specializes in health and pet topics for leading national publications. She is the "Healthy Pets" columnist for *Prevention* magazine and the author of eight books. Home is Oceanside, California and she can be reached through her web site: www.byarden.com.

BUCK JONES—Humorous Illustrator
Studio in Des Moines, Iowa and can be reached through his web site: www.buckjonesillustrator.com.

TABLE OF CONTENTS

Dr. Dale Anderson

AGELESS ALLIES

APPENDICES   101

INTRODUCTION

This book gives you permission to "act up" in good, happy, healthy ways.

Medical and pharmaceutical advances in the field of depression have helped millions become less sad, but not necessarily more happy. Researchers have found ways to turn off sadness but they are still searching for effective, healthy ways to "turn ON" happiness.

Too often, social, academic and scientific wisdom teaches that if we eliminate the negative we can accentuate the positive. This conventional thinking seems to miss a vital piece in the "puzzle of life." It's backwards. In reality, "accentuating the positive eliminates the negative."

When I entered the profession of medicine 45 years ago, the understanding of a physician's role was to help the sick regain good health. Doctors treated sick patients. Period! There was little or no attention given to the mind-body connection as it related to being ill or well. I could set broken limbs, give medicines to fight infection, and help patients heal following surgeries. If a pill or surgery wasn't helpful then the illness was often viewed as untreatable.

In time, however, it became clear to practitioners that the actions and thoughts of a person profoundly impacted their health. Sad and angry folks seem to be more prone to illness and self-abusive behavior. Happy folks seem to be healthier and respond faster to medical care. It became so obvious. Not only did health accentuate happiness, BUT, happiness accentuated health.

As did laughter! Do people laugh because they're happy? Or are they happy because they laugh? The answer is "YES," to both. The science of psycho-neuro-immunity confirms that those in UPbeat roles can elevate their feel-good chemistries and get into happy, healthy moods. Proof positive that feeling good is more than just not feeling bad.

What evokes happiness—and consequently, good health? Stable relationships, faithful friendships, loving families—caring for others and

Dr. Dale Anderson

being cared for by others. So does security, hope, self-confidence, spirituality, certain colors, aromas, plants, music—and for many, the unconditional love of a pet.

AND NOW, for those who need a fun "jumpstart"—Heeeeeeer's METHOD acting to help you INNERtain a WELLderly role that will turn ON the chemistry to look, think and feel younger—to be more childlike.

Never Act Your Age raises the curtain and shines the spotlight on ways to be a starring V.P. (Vintage Person). This book knocks the "EL" out of __derly. And prompts the debut of WELLderly headliners. This is where the ACT enters the scene. The science of acting and the art of healing when orchestrated in concert can add life to one's years and years to one's life.

You will discover that this book plays UP many unique ways to get "your WELLderly ACT together."

So don't be surprised when the doctor's orders—

- tell you to—"FAKE IT! 'til you make it," or
- dispense—a LAUGHTER PRESCRIPTION, or
- tell you— what to "stand UP for," or
- show how—J'ARMing is more fun than you can "shake a stick at," or
- preview—the revolutionary LIQUIDATION Diet for the WAIST-FULL

I, a physician nearing the 7th decade, am grateful every day to be the steward of the divine gift of life, a shared miraculous gift that is ours to play out WEll-aged.

I am honored to be designated as the AGED SAGE of the VINTAGE STAGE. And privileged to have you as a friend and patient-reader of this book!

And now! It's SHOW TIME!
Enjoy dramatic benefits.
Put on a happy face and
laugh for the "Health of IT."

Curtain UP! You're ON!

Dr. Dale Anderson

ACT 1

SET THE STAGE

A Historical Look at Acting WELL

As a physician with more than 40 years of medical practice, I've seen patients in this Theater of Life get into many different acts. I've seen young people act old. Old people act young. Well people act sick. And sick people act well. In each instance, these patients have "put ON" and "pulled OFF" great character IN-ACTments. Each has been able to get into the "chemistry of their part."

Regrettably, some folks became stuck in a painful, unhappy character role. Others, however, became shining stars who put on a happy face and played it UP. With rehearsal and practice, they created a pleasing, REAL classy act that they and others applauded and enjoy.

My diagnosis: people who positively script, stage, costume, direct and ACT happy, healthy and stress-free can actually change their body chemistry for the better. This INNER-taining performance compliments and enhances conventionally prescribed medications and treatments. Every doctor agrees that happy people are healthier. You might say, "they've got their act together—WELL!"

"All the world's a stage, and every man [and woman] merely players. We have our exits and our entrances and one person in their time plays many parts."

WILLIAM SHAKESPEARE

Theater and medicine? Strangely, yes, these two fields are intertwined. Together, the science of acting and the art of healing CAN add life to your years AND years to your life.

Must you suddenly audition for your community's next play? Try to land a walk-on part in Woody Allen's next movie? Or recite scenes from Shakespeare's *As You Like It* to your family before heading off to work each morning? NO.

But, you can ACT years younger than your actual age without ever having to take a step on an actual stage. When you're feeling sad, pessimistic, lethargic or overwhelmed, your body chemistry is different than when you're feeling happy, optimistic, energized, or in control. That's because **feelings are chemicals and chemicals are feelings.**

Yes, every feeling—sometimes called a mood, a state, or an emotion—has its own identifiable physiology. Therefore, this "chemistry" can become scientifically understood. And, these emotional chemistries can be changed by using acting techniques that get us moving, speaking, and thinking in different ways. You can truly be INNER-taining.

> **AGEless Wisdom**
>
> Happiness is a skill that takes practice.

The Scientific Roots of Acting Well

So, is this concept new? No, in fact, you may be surprised to learn that "acting UP" is actually centuries old. Some late greats in the fields of theater and medicine have helped scores of folks live—to die youthfully happy—at an old age; to die young, old.

English playwright William Shakespeare was but one of the theater healers to help folks get their acts together. Will certainly had a wonderful way with words. And, his words spoken on stage conveyed important life lessons. Shakespeare was savvy. He knew that

> **AGEless Wisdom**
>
> To grin and share it.

people actually occupy many stages in the course of their everyday lives. He knew that the dynamics of theater and life overlap.

Let's fast forward to the early 1900s and shine our spotlight on Constantin Stanislavski. Not exactly a household name like Shakespeare, but Stanislavski earns my top billing as a patron saint not only of the stage, but of health. Who was he? Stanislavski was an early 20th century Russian actor, director and

> ## AGEless Wisdom
> We don't laugh because we're happy—we're happy because we laugh.

teacher of actors. He belonged to the prestigious Moscow Arts Theatre during the time of the Bolshevik Revolution. He has been called Russia's finest actor, but his legacy comes from the creation of a system of acting so well known that it is often simply referred to as "The Method." (See Stanislavski quotes in the Appendix)

Stanislavski was years ahead of his time with his understanding of the mind-body connection. He taught actors how to evoke believable emotions on stage—and to do so with conviction. His villains appeared and FELT truly vile and villainous; heroes were heartwarmingly heroic. Tears and laughter poured out so fully and freely from the actors that the audience became IN-TRANCED with the physiology being TRANCE-ACTED on stage.

Stanislavski modified his technique throughout his life and earned recognition as being one of the most influential contributors to theater science.

Think of your favorite movie stars and why you applaud their stellar performances. "Everyman" Oscar-winning actor Tom Hanks appears to be a chocolate-loving simple man named Forrest Gump in one movie and then a clever hero in *Apollo 13*. He then convinces us that he can conduct conversations with a volleyball named Wilson on a desert island and in another movie, lead a World War II platoon in search of an Army private named Ryan.

I am certain that Stanislavski's Method helps actors modify their physiology on stage by teaching them how to tap into the chemistry of anger, sadness, happiness, and all the other feelings required in roles of the characters they played. And his technique continues to assist actors to time those TRANCE-formations in chemistries on cue—at the precise moment that these feelings are called for on stage.

But his Method is not limited to actors on stage. His technique can also help you and I change our emotional chemistry on cue at the precise moments when these feelings are needed. When we act WELL, we create a more satisfying role on the stage of daily life.

"Stan the Man" identified physical, mental and staging strategies for effective acting. He trained his acting students to produce an emotional-chemical response to get into their roles.

Stanislavski came up with an astounding equation that is right on the mark:

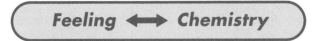

Feeling ⟷ Chemistry

For your *Never Act Your Age* role, let's look at his categories that determine chemistry and feelings:

Physical: When you "enter" into the character role you want to play—that is, to be a happier, more UPbeat person, you need to make appropriate changes in your posture, walk, gestures and especially the face you wear. And don't overlook basic health practices such as hygiene, nutrition, breathing, and exercise.

Mental: To get into the desired mood, you need to make changes in thinking, beliefs, images and self-dialogue. That requires doing some education and scripting.

Stage: It is vital that you "set the stage" by paying attention to scenery, props, costume lighting, sounds, smells, and your personal supporting cast—those 3Ps: people, pets and plants in your daily drama.

The PHYSICAL, MENTAL, STAGE

PHYSICAL
Nutrition
Hygiene
Breathing
Exercise
Posture
Gesture
Walk

MENTAL
Thoughts
Beliefs
Imaging
Self-Dialogue
Scripting
Education

FEELING ⟷ CHEMISTRY

STAGE
Props
Scenery
Costume
Senses—light, smell, sound, touch,
temperature
3P's—People, Pets, Plants

© Copyright: Dale L. Anderson, M.D., J'ARM, Inc.

5

Stanislavski didn't limit his circle of colleagues to thespians. He had scientific associates. In a strange but wonderful introduction between theater and science, Stanislavski headed to St. Petersburg to meet the famed physiologist named Ivan Pavlov. This Russian scientist earned the Nobel Prize (with a bell) in 1904 for his series of studies involving the digestive systems of dogs.

Pavlov discovered that if he rang a bell each time he fed dogs, the dogs would associate the bell with food. Eventually, he noted that the dogs began to salivate each time they heard the bell ring— even when their food bowls were empty. His experiments proved that the dogs had been *conditioned* to secrete digestive juices at the sound of the bell. He discovered how to manipulate and trigger a specific type of inner chemistry.

Stanislavski thought Pavlov was a real dog-gone good guy.

I've often wished that I could have witnessed the meeting of these creative minds. Permit me a little literary license as I recap how their initial conversations might have gone:

"You know, Dr. Pavlov, when I heard about your tests with dogs, I was upset at first. It's kind of a cheap trick to make those poor dogs think they're going to get food and then just ring a bell in their faces. That's changing their chemistry by trickery."

Stanislavski then makes a dramatic pause before continuing:

"I got to thinking, Ivan, about what you're doing and I started wondering whether I could do something with my acting students that is very much like what you're doing with your dogs. Is there a way of getting my acting students to *put on the dog?* Now, I don't want to make my students salivate at the sound of a bell, but I am seeking a way to trigger a chemical and physical response in my students—an emotional response that will help them perform on stage and that will be felt by the audience."

To which Pavlov may have responded, "My good comrade, Constantin. You'll be *pawsitively* pleased to know that you don't have to treat your students like dogs! You are right in recognizing that there is a definite connection between physiology and the actions and thoughts of every human behavior."

Learn How to Change Your Act

When we keep performing a role over and over again, it becomes part of a living physiology. Eventually, the chemistry of that ACT becomes so believable that it is reinforced by all of those around us. They treat us according to how we ACT and then the chemistry does indeed, become REAL.

Remember Audrey Hepburn in the movie classic *My Fair Lady?* In her role, she transformed a low-on-the-social-rung Eliza Doolittle into the Belle of the Ball, thanks to lots of directing by Professor Higgins. Scene after scene, everything about her ACT changed, from her posture, her clothing, how she walked and how she talked (*the rain in Spain falls mainly on the plain—by jove, she's got it!*).

While under the tutelage of Professor Higgins, Eliza still didn't quite have the inner chemistry that felt real. It wasn't until she was TREATED and RECOGNIZED as having these qualities by a wealthy, slick Hungarian at the social ball. The Hungarian treated her as a lady and called her a lady. And it was THEN that her physiology transformed, enabling her to feel like the "real" person she had become—a lady—for the first time.

There's even a psychological term for this type of transformation: The Pygmalion Effect.

> **Lesson learned: if you act well, people will treat you like you are well. Conversely, when you act sick, people will treat you like you are sick. And, when you act old, people will treat you like you're old and when you act young, people will treat you like you're young—you choose!**

It is your act AND your audience's acceptance of your performance that create your REAL chemistry.

Norman Cousins
Adopts and Adapts the Endorphins

Another personal, happy hero of mine was Norman Cousins. His 1979 bestseller, *Anatomy of an Illness*, spotlighted and popularized the scientific field of mind-body medicine called psychoneuroimmunology (PNI). Don't let the size of that word daunt you. To gain a true understanding of the word, just break it down into three parts:

Psycho—refers to mental processes including thoughts, beliefs, mental images, and feelings.

Neuro—refers to the chemistry of the nervous system (the brain and the spinal cord) as well as hormones that regulate emotions.

Immunology—refers to the body's ability to resist disease and various types of infection.

Cousins explored this vital link between feeling and healing, mind and body. He had plenty of internal motivation.

As editor of the *Saturday Review*, Cousins suffered from ankylosing spondylitis, a painful, degenerative disease that can be fatal. But Cousins was an unconventional, creative healer. He took a more active role in his medical treatment by moving his hospital bed into a nearby hotel room. There, he created a cozy, home-like environment and paid attention to his mental and emotional states. He saw the medicinal value in viewing classic comedy films such as Laurel and Hardy and TV programs like *Candid Camera*.

Guess what? His health dramatically improved.

Let's let him explain:

"I made the joyous discovery that 10 minutes of genuine belly laughter had an anesthetic effect and would give me at least two hours of pain-free sleep."

In time, Cousins no longer needed medications. He had become completely cured of ankylosing spondylitis. But Cousins was no selfish guy. He quit the magazine and joined the staff at UCLA Medical School in Los Angeles where he continued his mission to probe and study the field of PNI with top physicians and researchers.

Did Cousins merely laugh himself to good health? That would be too simplistic of a response. I say that Cousins used laughter AND other fun "feel good," positive ACTS. His holistic medicine was wisely blended and teamed with conventional medicine. This man significantly contributed to the understanding of why a wise, happy role "plays out" WELL.

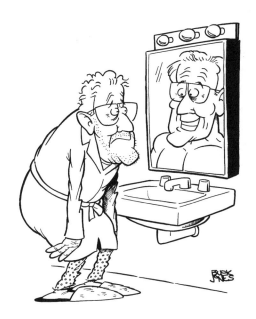

Norman Cousins wrote about his impressive recovery, "laughter probably played a part to release endorphins." Soon, he and other researchers working in the field of PNI began to refer to all the beneficial "feel good" neurotransmitter chemicals—broadly—as endorphins. For the non-scientific community, the term has become "generic" and encompasses not only the "honest to goodness" endorphins, but all of their respectable shirt-tail relatives. The ENDO(inner) (m)ORPHINS are often called the inner uppers that get us "high on life."

My Patient Offers Good Advice

I credit an actress patient of mine for helping me truly realize how the chemistry of the performing arts can impact health. You might say that she "opened the curtain" for me into this mind-body connection. She helped me realize that it was not just actors who perform. Everyone is on the stage of life every day. We all need to get into the chemistry of our desired roles.

During each office visit for a period of several months, this actress would complain of different aches and pains. Thorough exams and diagnostic tests could not explain these symptoms. No treatment approach—medication, physical therapy—seemed to work. Then one day, EUREKA! The clue to her ailing was revealed.

Propped on the exam table wearing an expression of pain, the actress asked, "Could it be the part?" She tearfully continued. "I can't live as the person I've become. I'm playing a hateful, disgusting character on stage and this 'witchy' role stays with me 24 hours a day. It's an angry, uptight, wretched part. IT'S A PAINFUL PART."

And then the most provocative question I have ever had from a patient!

She sobbed, "Could the chemistry of this role be bad for my health? Is the chemistry of this sick role being played out—in illness and pain?"

The answer to that question and the treatment of her problems were soon obvious.

WOW! Within a few weeks when the "painful" play had its final curtain call, she auditioned and won the role of an UPbeat character in a comedy classic. Soon she was playing a happy part WELL—both on stage and off. The old chemistry of the sickening witch had been "washed out of her system." The stage was re-set. An INNERtaining new bio-physiology emerged and her health improved dramatically.

Coincidence? NO! It was the chemistry, the "nature" of the happy role. My actress patient had successfully managed to create a new chemical mood that felt good, and soon felt REAL.

On her last visit, she nearly bounded off the exam table sporting an ear-to-ear grin and bright dancing eyes: "You know, Doctor Dale, in any part, you have to be there before you're there. You have to INact a specific chemistry of a character's emotion before you are believable. You must act and think the part over and over and over again until it becomes REAL."

"Like forming a habit?" I offered. "Like a Pavlovian Response?"

"That's IT!" she exclaimed. "With practice, everyone can get their act together."

Bravo!

Dr. Seuss Rallies Good Health

One of my favorite authors who has helped me get my act together and who has set the stage to help thousands of VPs (Vintage People) and kids of all ages was and is Dr. Seuss. He knew how to turn on happy, healthy feelings with his wonderful rhymes. To this day, I enjoy reading his *Green Eggs and Ham* to my grandchildren.

So, let's end this ACT 1 chapter and put a smile on your face by sharing an excerpt from Dr. Seuss' book, *Oh, the Places You'll Go!:*

Congratulations!
Today is your day.
You're off to Great Places!
You're off and away!
You have brains in your head.
You have feet in your shoes.
You can steer yourself
Any direction you choose.

So be sure when you step.
Step with care and great tact
and remember that Life's
a Great Balancing Act.

I hope that this all-star cast from Shakespeare to Stanislavski to Pavlov to Cousins to Seuss and to my actress patient will IN-courage and IN-able your performance on this earthly stage to be one of fun, pleasure, delight, love, health and happiness. I hope that with your INNER-taining chemistry humming, you will IN-joy a life that's a smash hit. A long-running hit! A life-long hit—heralded with much applause, many bravos and rave reviews. And when the final curtain falls, all will celebrate, and say, "This was a performance WELL done!"

BRAVO!

Ageless Ally

After more than three decades as a high school football coach and a drama teacher, Ert Jones-Hermerding will retire soon.

He enters this new phase of his life without a playbook or a script. Intentionally.

"I could continue to teach, but there are other things I want to do and need to do. I view my so-called retirement with excitement—it is not a negative. I will re-invent myself and I can't wait to re-fire," says Jones-Hermerding of Plymouth, Minnesota.

He has spent a lifetime re-inventing himself and loving every minute of it.

As a new graduate looking for a teaching job, well-meaning mentors suggested that he must choose an either-or path: football or theater. No one can coach football AND direct student plays while being a classroom teacher.

"I decided to buck stereotyping and pursue both of my passions," he said. "I tell my students that good, caring people can taint your opinion, they can shatter your confidence. You've got to believe in yourself. If you're not passionately committed internally, nothing you do will work."

Just as Jones-Hermerding was hitting his stride as a winning football coach, he again broke with tradition. He sidelined himself for five years to spend more time with his young children, Harper and Meelynn, and his wife, Pat, who is also a teacher.

"I wanted to watch them grow up, and it was a difficult decision to temporarily leave coaching, but I knew it was the right one," he says. "I discovered that the kids were energizing me. I found myself laughing a great deal."

His lesson he now passes on to younger coaches with families: "take two years off and you will not regret it. And it will make you a better coach. I know it did me."

"And, as a teacher, I'm a role model—a job I take very seriously. I strive to teach kids how to learn to live their lives by watching positive, happy, energized people."

Ert Jones-Hermerding

Dr. Dale Anderson

Turn ON the
"CHEMISTRY"
Tune UP the Music

I love parades featuring marching bands. The synchronized marching steps. The trumpets harmonizing with the flutes. The drums tapping the beat. It's teamwork at its best.

In many ways, you have a marching band performing inside your body. And leading this band of good-doers are the endorphins, chemicals called the "inner uppers." In step and following close behind are lines and lines of the finest virtuosos, the other UPbeat neuropeptides. Together, in harmony, these chemicals turn ON the "high notes" of our happy inner music. This band of do-gooders is the natural chemistry of our bodies that get us HIGH on life.

And self-medicating with them is easy. All you need to do is get in line and play the happy part. Play UP your actions and your thoughts. In other words, get in step with the A.C.T. Approach (Action, Chemistry and Thought). Method actors know

"The human race has only one effective weapon, and that's laughter. The moment it arises, all our hardnesses yield, all our irritations and resentments slip away, and a sunny spirit takes their place."

MARK TWAIN

that emotional chemistry is generated through actions and thoughts. Thus the acronym A.C.T. Now!

Actions get us into a chemistry and thoughts get us into a chemistry, but what is also true is that actions can get us into thoughts and

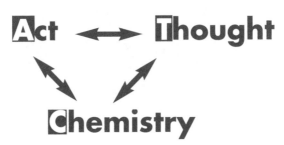

thoughts can get us into actions. They are all inter-related. This equation works in all directions! Actions, Thoughts and Chemistry are INtricately INtwined.

As a conventionally trained physician and board-certified HOLIS-TIC practitioner, I am often the designer, director, producer, conductor and coach of many healing events. But not the star. Because I am not on stage or on the playing field. The patient is! But over the years, it has become apparent that the success of those on stage is dramatically improved if they and their coaches recognize that life is SHOW BUSINESS. We are all in our act and we are all role models.

I take great pride in prescribing theater techniques that help my patients-friends. And now you, helping you get your act together, to set your stage and to live a happy, healthy part—WELL. It's an honor to help you perfect your new role, to INact a youthful, ageless, WELLderly part.

Make Method Acting a Holistic Healer

In fact, your INactment will help identify Method Acting as the "holistic medicine" of the 21st century. No question about it, you can become healthier and happier and more successful by consciously staging, scripting, costuming, and acting the part of a successful, happy, energetic, contented, and healthy person who lives life to the fullest. By doing so, you turn on the chemistry that promotes WELL being and feeling good.

And, the best part: medical science can measure qualitatively and quantitatively the chemistry of feelings. These feelings can even be pictured on brain PET scans (Positron Emission Topography). A graphic depiction can

> ### AGEless Wisdom
>
> Adopt an
> ENDORPHIN.

show the map of different feelings and emotions within a person. In fact, a PET scan can HIGHlight when and where the chemistry of happiness is turned ON. The PET scan is a shining example of how happy emotions can brighten up the brain. And, in turn, brighten us up and INlighten the world.

So, let's learn about your body's chemistry. I guarantee no lectures, term papers, or final exams!

Ready? Class is now in session!

Let's start with a l-o-n-g word: psychoneuroimmunology. A quick refresher definition from ACT 1: PNI deals with the connection between the nervous system (the body's boss for memory and emotion), the endocrine system (the warehouse for powerful hormones), and the immune system (the body's internal army against microbial invasions).

Now Starring: Endorphins

Endorphins are just one branch of the PNI neuropeptide family. But they merit marquee-like attention. Endorphins are in-body versions of morphine. Like morphine, endorphins can fight pain, but at strengths 200 to 2,000 times MORE powerful than morphine and WITHOUT any nasty side effects. Endorphins can prevent certain brain cells from transmitting impulses, giving endorphins the power to block pain and to produce feelings of euphoria.

Here is a list of not one or two but TEN ways these feel-good endorphins and neuropeptides can cast you into the role of happy, more youthful health:

1. Ease aches and pain
2. Relax tensed muscles
3. Calm fears
4. Tone down anger
5. Suppress the appetite
6. Lessen depression
7. Decrease inflammation
8. Boost your immune system
9. Generate euphoric WELLbeing
10. Enhance a longer, healthier life

But that's not all! Endorphins and the "happy" neuropeptides are SOCIAL turn-ons, too. Folks who tap into their INNER UPPERS are often more:

1. Popular (leaders of the band)
2. Attractive (rarely have a bad hair day)
3. Skillful
4. Energetic
5. Inquisitive
6. Teachable—learn new skills easily
7. Creative and perceptive
8. Confident and courageous
9. Optimistic
10. Physically active
11. Youthful
12. Wealthy

These two lists show that the chemistry of successful health, wealth and happiness appears to be related. Now that's one chemical family whom I'd like to be a-kin to. And many WELLderly already are! But for those who are not yet in this happy clan, it's time to MERRY UP with those who are.

> **AGEless Wisdom**
>
> Grinners are Winners.

Warning! Watch out! Don't allow draining, negative "show stoppers" bring down your endorphin lights and shut the curtain on your opportunity to play IT UP.

Now, let's look at how endorphins and their supporting cast of happy neuropeptides perform their roles. When we laugh, feel good, exercise or get joy from cuddling with our partner or a pet, our cells release good-feeling chemistries. At the same time, other cells (lymphocytes, T-cells, Natural Killer cells, and macrophages) and chemicals like gamma globulins are increased. Body chemicals such as cortisol decrease.

These cells and chemicals represent the body's immune squad that seeks and destroys invading bacteria and viruses. And, if we could take a peek at the energy activity, we would see a lot of fireworks—millions of tiny explosive reactions. These cells fire off electrical I-ONic charges, thus communicating via chemicals to other nerve cells, muscle and organ tissues.

Like the marching band, the orchestration of these chemical charges results in the delivery of messages that are played out to the rest of the body. And, this INNER music affects our actions, our thoughts and our emotions. Our motions, notions and emotions are all regulated by our chemistries.

Remember that the A.C.T. equation flows ALL directions between the A, the C and the T components of our HOLISTIC acting! (See diagram on page 16). What's the happy result of all this harmonizing? Marching in step with the rest of the band provides a happy harmony that connects us to ourselves and to others so that we all feel (chemistry) great.

Oliver Wendell Holmes said, "What a pity so many people die with their music in them."

But now, we can wonder if it isn't even a greater tragedy that so many in our society do not realize that all of us are born with happy chemical music within—just waiting to be enjoyed. There is always time to tune UP, turn ON and to strike UP the band to appreciate the high notes played OUT when we perform the happy, WELL-derly role with dramatic flare.

Fake It—Doctor's Orders!

AGEless Wisdom

Put your funny
where your
mouth is.

Yes, fake it! Fake it! Fake it! Fake it! 'Til ya make IT! And guess what happens? Even "fake" laughter can cue the cells into releasing the endorphin-related chemicals. Fake them UP and you're on your way to a happier and healthier outlook. Yes, raising endorphins is just an ACT. By merely ACTING UPbeat, you reap the benefits of your internal pharmacy. It is open 24 hours a day to cater to your needs. To get the prescription filled, however, you must have the key that opens this cellular pharmacy. And the key is to A.C.T.

Putting ON happy Actions opens the INNER pharmacy. Merely thinking UP an UPPER notion or believing that a medication or a treatment works can raise endorphins and related chemicals. This is an example of pos-I-tive Actions and Thinking being used to promote a dramatic INprovement in health.

What? You say you're in a blue mood? Or feeling a bit achy? Oh, too bad!

The solution may be to take some "imaginary placebo medicine."

Yes, choose to "fake some good feelings" until the new chemistry feels real. Fake it! Fake it! Fake it! 'Til ya make IT! If you have nothing to smile about, fake a smile, fake laughter. Pretend to be happy and start

ACTing like you are. Just stand in front of the mirror each morning and belly laugh for 15 seconds. (Rehearse the Laughter Rx in Act 4 on page 58.)

Laugh for the sheer HEALTH of IT!

Laughter, whether REAL or FAKE, creates a chemistry that makes people happy and thereby promotes good health. There is a definite mind-body connection at play here.

Just as downer emotions and mood affect our immune system negatively, so can our upper emotions, moods, actions and thoughts affect our immune system positively. We can't have any thoughts or actions without a predictable physiology resulting. Actions and thoughts can fire UP a happy chemistry. And quite naturally, a happy chemistry can fire UP happy actions and thoughts. Remember that all feelings are chemistry and chemistry is feelings. They are one and the same. The A.C.T. is never-ending. And, the happy

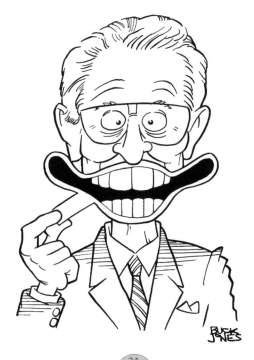

A.C.T. can be successfully performed as an UPbeat, long-running HIT (Review Physical, Mental, Stage Diagram on page 5 in ACT 1).

The scientific field of psychoneuroimmunology yields a host of insights about measurable physiological links between emotional levels and overall health. Research has proven time and time again that a good, happy, UPbeat WELLderly role evokes increased levels of AGE-less endorphins and related chemicals. They call this positive state "eustress." And let me stress that pleasurable YOUstress is what keeps the energized WELLderly UP and running. BUT—

That said. We need to read the fine print and look at the flip side to all of this. One of the "villains" in the "This Is Your Life" play is negative stress. It's inescapable in today's "must do, got-to be-here, got-to-be-there" world. But, it can be controlled. Countless studies have shown that negative stress creates unhealthy physiological changes in your body. There's a direct connection between stressful stress and muscle tension, high blood pressure, headaches, and a weakened immune system. The list goes on—stress can aggravate a wide range of problems, from dandruff, hair loss, and acne to diarrhea, constipation, and hives. Get stressed about anything and the condition will likely get worse.

When we get S-T-R-E-S-S-E-D, the adrenal glands open the gate and release corticosteroids, which quickly convert to cortisol in the blood stream. This raised cortisol and other chemical villains suppress your immune system, making you more vulnerable to disease. The big concern: the incident that is causing you stress doesn't have to be real. The mere PERCEPTION of a threat is enough to send your chemical stress level soaring. The belief becomes true. Becomes real.

But, the A.C.T. approach INables one to YOUstress the chemistry of a positive part. And to play it WELL!

Here are eight Physiological "Downers" that can close a "show" before it even opens:

1. Poor physical condition
2. Poor posture
3. Poor sleep
4. Poor finances (Poor fiscal shape)
5. Chronic pain
6. Pain medications
7. Chronic stress
8. Negative, complaining "nay" sayers

Laugh Negative Stress Away

Looking for an antidote—a free one—for negative stress and other unhealthy "villains"? Oh course! One of the easiest and most simple antidotes to INact is laughter. Yes, the whole gamut from chuckles and giggles to full-belly guffaws can be handy self-care tools to shoo away negative feelings. Let these joyous expressions step UP and "set the stage" for dramatic improvements in your health. Laughter lowers elevated cortisol levels and encourages your immune system to behave more efficiently.

Fortunately, physicians and patients are understanding and talking more about the mind-body connection. Dean Ornish, M.D., a cardiologist, is also the best-selling author of *Dr. Dean Ornish's Program for Reversing Heart Disease*. In his book, he demonstrated that people can actually REVERSE the effects of heart disease by making healthy lifestyle changes that include low-fat diets, regular exercise, stress management, and getting AND giving social support.

Many conventional medical schools and medical centers are creating stress reduction clinics that incorporate meditation in treating people with chronic pain. Oncologists, infectious disease specialists, and physicians who treat chronic health problems are becoming cheerleaders for INacting the endorphins.

Elevated endorphin levels play vital roles in improving the healing and survival rates of their patients.

We are still learning new ways to blend conventional and "unconventional" health care approaches together to bolster our immunity. We now recognize that by tapping into the mind-body connection, we can reap measurable results in the chemistry of healing. By incorporating the study of acting techniques, we can also learn how to think the right thoughts and make the right moves to evoke the beneficial chemistry of healing.

It's NOT the Same OLD A.C.T. Anymore!

I passionately believe that the theater techniques for the happy part should be identified and played out on the stage of everyday life. That's why the A.C.T. Now Project and the A.C.T Now Foundation serve as the catalyst that will prompt

"the dramatic arts to think medically and
the medical arts to think dramatically."

The A.C.T. approach will become the HOLISTIC medicine of the 21st century. And when it does, the dramatic benefits will be contagious.

WELLderly "stars" like you and other "happy players" of all ages are getting their A.C.T.s together. And as more like you and I understand how to set the INNER chemistry of joy, love, and laughter, a healthy, infectious, HAPPYdemic will spread. Worldwide. Then, hopefully, together, every person will play out a happy part—WELL-aged.

DRAMATIC!
BRAVO!

Ageless Ally

Patty Wooten, R.N., walks into the hospital ward. The eyes of the patients focus not on her nametag, or the stethoscope hanging around her neck. They see the big, brilliant red ball that covers her nose. Some smile. Many break out in infectious laughter.

Wooten, age 55, of Santa Cruz, California, has helped patients, their relatives and medical staffs mend and heal physically—and emotionally—for more than 30 years. Since 1976, she has bolstered her bedside manner by offering the therapeutic powers of laughter as a professional clown.

"My nursing and clowning came together partly by accident and partly as a result of a low time in my life," says Wooten, now a renowned international speaker often referred to as the "Queen of Jest."

But back in 1976, her life was in turmoil; she was newly divorced, trying to raise her young son, Ken. Her job was one of constant life and death decisions. Money was tight. Her emotions were tense.

"Then, on my way to work one day, I heard an ad on my car radio about a clown school. I remember the words: 'How would you like to make others laugh?' I thought to myself that here was a chance to do something that would take me away from the seriousness of life."

Wooten enrolled and became "Curly the Clown." Clown school taught her how to tap her true "inner clown" and to take more of a childlike—not childish—attitude toward life.

Soon she started to study and has since become an expert on the serious, therapeutic side of humor and how laughter can improve a person's physical health and mental outlook.

Today she rarely pays attention to her chronological age. She feels ageless because her life is shaped by sharing with others how they can "tickle their funny bone." How they can create and enjoy the benefits of laughter.

"All of us have a pent-up need to laugh. Find what makes you laugh and who you laugh the most with and you will feel healthier and happier," she says.

Patty Wooten, R.N.

ACT

STAGE ENERGY
Handle "BITE" Parts WELL

Folks, the idea of aging is changing. Growing older no longer automatically means we're growing OLD or becoming ANCIENT. We are actually living longer—and better—because we are learning how to "right" our scripts for healthier lives.

Getting the best out of life means being willing to keep learning and growing. Thoughts of the old status quo simply have to go! Don't be stuck in an old mindset or an old habit so deeply that you are never open to good change, to progress, to becoming WELLderly.

I, for example, am a traditionally trained medical doctor who has "practiced" for more than 40 years as a board-certified surgeon, board-certified emergency physician and board-certified HOLISTIC Medicine physician. I still practice as a Medicare-Card-Carrying doctor by caring for patients in the Urgent Care Clinics of a large health care group in the Twin Cities Metro area of Minnesota.

While I celebrate the wonderful advances of conventional medicine, I also embrace the many healing powers of HOLISTIC medicine. When blended well, conventional and HOLISTIC medicines work as a wonderful team to get us healthy.

"Age is simply a number. More is better."
ANONYMOUS

For years, patients have asked me what herbs, vitamins, minerals, aromas and mind-body approaches they should use to augment their blood pressure prescriptions. They wanted to know what foods would help reduce their risks for developing cancer, heart disease, or pain. In short, they were looking for all the "little tricks" that when taken together, could set the stage for a WELLderly role. They were looking for simple, easy-to-follow natural suggestions that *work*.

I use the following techniques to keep myself childlike (not childish) as my seventh decade nears. For more than 25 years, I have wanted to better understand all the health approaches often referred to as "alternative medicine." My desire was to listen with no preconceived "scientific" bias, no desire to embrace or to discredit. I merely wanted to understand what my patients were finding healing and beneficial in "Grandma's Remedies" or other mind/body health practices and beliefs.

So, despite sporting a head full of silver hair, I knew I was never too old to go back to school. I enrolled in osteopathic manipulation and other HOLISTIC medicine courses to learn about the healing powers of herbs, nutrition, supplements, meditation, body manipulation, homeopathy and more. And, in 2001, at age 68, I became board certified by the American Board of Holistic Medicine.

In essence, I "righted" my script as a physician and discovered what many shamanistic healers and grandmas and grandpas have known for centuries as "good medicine." And when this healing "wisdom" is blended with conventional medicine, the integration of the two provides multiple benefits.

You can right your script, too. Set yourself for the performance of your life by starting with what's on your dinner plate. Let me show you how you CAN take a bite out of aging. The right quantity and quality of foods CAN extend your life. The right supplements and herbs CAN help you feel more youthful and childlike.

The Liquidation Diet©

is a splash hit

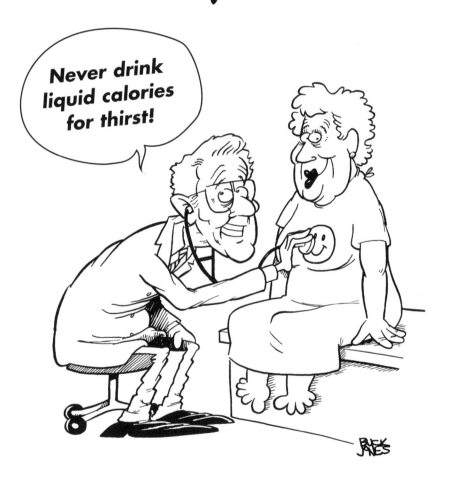

Take a Bite Out of Aging

Explorer Ponce de Leon searched in vain for the elusive Fountain of Youth along the northeast coast of Florida five centuries ago. Still today, we are always searching to find something that will add to our good health.

In fact, you need only to stroll to your refrigerator or food pantry or, better yet, AWAY from your refrigerator or food pantry—to accomplish your quest for feeling young. When you are about to eat or drink, WAIT. And WEIGHT.

Sixty percent of the USA population is overweight. That has become a HUGE health problem for our country. For those who are BIG STARS, the show gets out early. How many overweight people do you see who are in their eighth decade?

What do you have to lose? Extra pounds are often the behind-the-scenes culprit contributing to diabetes, hypertension, and heart problems and pain and muscle weakness. Being overloaded with too much "fr-weight" contributes to almost all orthopedic problems, especially pain, and stiffness in the back and lower extremities.

As I tell many patients, "You can't drive a Mac truck on Volkswagen tires. Soooooo, I say, "Take it off. Take it off!" Tastefully, slowly and sensibly.

What I don't emphasize is the word, D-I-E-T. The word "diet" is too often interpreted to mean deprivation, punishment, and failure. Diet's true meaning is derived from its Greek root, meaning simply— "a way of life."

Every year, we are bombarded by "new" and "breakthrough" diets that promise to melt away pounds almost overnight. They come and go! Come and go! The list of diets includes high/low protein or high/low fat or high/low carbohydrates or one-food diets like grapefruit, bananas or popcorn—even pizza. It is a never-ending cast of diets—spawning many sequels. Clinic after clinic, plan after plan—most pitching programs that "suggest the purchase of a formulated supplements and/or packaged, nutritionally balanced meals." The truth is that too many diets have been touted and EATEN UP by people anxious to find an EASY "MELT DOWN." All too often these authors or "Clinic Managers" are self-appointed nutritional experts who hope to FATTEN their bank accounts at the EXPANSE of their readers and clients. In essence, diet authors are making a living from your "liquid" assets.

Let's stop this foolishness. If you are overweight, liquidate now. Here is the only "diet book" that you will ever need. And, it's just a few pages long. It's an easy "way of life" to follow! It's called The Liquidation Diet.

Never drink liquid calories for thirst.

There, in a mere six words, is The Liquidation Diet. And it will help you painlessly shed WAIST-FULL pounds if you are overweight.

Let me explain. If you eliminate *all* caloric drinks—with the exception of a judicious glass of red wine at a festive occasion—

Here's a handy list of drinks that can easily be LIQUIDATED

with their estimated approximate calories.

4–6 ounces of juice = 100 to 120 calories
8 ounces of milk = 100 to 150 calories
16 ounces of a "sports drink" = 100–150 calories
12 ounces of soda = 120 calories
12 ounces of beer = 100 to 130 calories

In a month, daily consumption can easily top 3,500 calories. And one pound of fat equals 3,500 calories.

---

you can lose a dozen or more pounds a year. Repeat: if you're overweight, don't swallow a liquid calorie from a cup, glass, can, or bottle.

Fruit and vegtable juice, soft drinks, athletic drinks, beer, cocktails, milk, and coffee or tea with cream or sugar are "waist-full" calories. If you drink one 8-ounce glass of milk a day, you ingest the caloric equivalent of one "fat" pound each month—more than 10 pounds in a year. The same holds true if you drink one can of soda or one small glass of juice a day. If you drink all three every day, you risk gaining three pounds a month—or 36 pounds in a single year! If you stop sipping and guzzling and make no other changes in your diet you will peel away over 36 pounds in a single year.

Let me share with you the story of an overweight, Type II diabetic, hypertensive patient with back and joint problems. He was a "juicer," who drank four glasses of juice, two glasses of milk, and 2 cans of sugared soda a day. And, he didn't exercise. Even if he kept all other aspects of his life constant and just "liquidated" his liquid habit, he could shed more than 80 pounds per year. Now, that's a showstopper! Fortunately, he heeded the advice to "liquidate" and his "juicy" weight peeled away. And his diabetes, hypertension and discomforts melted away as his fat came off painlessly.

Except for cooking needs and those times you want to be spoon-fed, I urge you to oust milk, juice, soda, sport drinks and beer from your refrigerator. Liquidate them out of your house. Liquidate them out of your life.

What do you drink instead? Do what I do. Drink 8 to 16 glasses of calorie-free water or tea for thirst every day. My coffee is black. I never sip a single calorie in liquid form—except for the occasional glass of "medicinal" red wine, a party beer or nonfat milk on my morning cereal. OK, well sometimes at bedtime a bit of "grandma's brandy." My liquid calories mostly come spoonful by spoonful as soup or as milk on cereal, but never gulped from a glass, cup, can or bottle.

If you follow this simple way of life—The Liquidation Diet—you, too, will become and remain a healthy "lightweight." Never again will you be swallowed in by fad diets.

The real skinny on looking younger is choosing a diet featuring these marquee headliners: whole grains, fruits, fish, lean meats, and green veggies. After all, food IS fuel. The healthy choices will reduce your risk of developing heart disease, stroke, diabetes, cancers, and obesity. And, by eating rather than drinking your fruits, you may even add 5, 10, or more productive, *fruitful* years to your life.

As we become VPs (Vintage People), our digestive systems tend be less than perfect performers. Eating habits, medications, and stress all influence how well our digestive system functions. Our taste and thirst buds become impaired and our stomachs secrete less hydrochloric acid and other digestive juices as we age. Certain medications, including aspirin, antibiotics, anti-inflammatories, and steroids can sometimes cause imbalances to the digestive system. With aging, some reduction of blood flow to the digestive tract can result in a reduced amount of nutrients being absorbed from the gut.

Vitamins and the minerals are vital to becoming WELLderly. As we age, our appetites tend to decrease naturally—but let's not let this blow us away. Being slightly underweight is good. Being skinny is not. Eating disorders that cause underweight conditions are a serious problem at any age. If a person is frail or underweight, eat and drink all the nutritious items you want—and more. But remember, a balanced lifestyle and diet is the answer.

Just like a successful theatrical production depends on its entire cast and stage crew to make the show a smashing success, your digestive system depends on multiple players to perform well.

Digest This: Easy Eating Tips

Sometimes, a simple change in your eating habits can do a world of good for your digestive system. Improve digestion by considering these helpful strategies:

Eat a generous breakfast.
> As the curtain of the day rises, a nutritious breakfast should be the first thing on your "playbill." Think protein and fiber.

Chew slowly.
> Your mom was right in nagging you to chew each bite of food. The one-bite-and-swallow eating style can cause big chunks of food to slow down your digestive process or worse—cause choking.

Close your mouth between sips and bites.
> The more air you swallow at mealtime, the greater the chance excess air will get trapped inside your stomach. The buildup of air can only be relieved by the expulsion of air—better known as the embarrassing belch. Or as the gastroenterologists tell me, the gas can be carried FART-HER and result in a noxious emission. "Butt" in the "end," the discomfort will pass.

Do the dinner plate comparison test.
> During a meal, check the plates of your eating companions. If your plate is empty and their plates are three-fourths full of food, that's your cue that you're eating *too fast*.

Turn off the TV.
> Instead of wolfing down food while watching your favorite sitcom, try paying more attention to the food and engage in friendly and *calm* conversation with your dinner mates. Avoid politics and religion as dinnertime topics.

If you're eating alone, read the paper.
Purposely turn the pages with the hand you hold a fork with so you are forced to put the fork down and slow down your chewing. Or, do the crossword puzzle or even better, read the comic page.

Take a hike—or at least a brisk 20- or 30-minute walk after—or before—dinner. Your strides go a long way in keeping your body toned and able to digest food better.

Salute your appetizer allies.
If you eat a salad or a cup of soup before the main course, you will be able to cut down on your caloric intake. Eating warm meals with a delicious aroma can actually cut down on food consumption, too.

Eat five small meals a day instead of three big ones.
Your body is able to digest smaller portions more easily than large meals.

Wait 20 minutes before dishing up seconds.
Your digestive system takes about 20 minutes to communicate with your brain the feeling of eating enough (*satiety*). Drink a glass of water between helpings and you may discover you're satisfied without seconds.

Eat more broccoli and broiled fish.
Green vegetables are great sources of fiber and essential nutrients. Fish provides the healthy omega fatty acids your body needs.

Avoid fats, especially animal fats and saturated vegetable fats, palm and coconut oils and trans-fatty oils.
The best oil choices are olive, walnut and canola oils.

Learn to share.
When you are eating at a restaurant, try splitting an entrée with a friend. Or, take half of your meal home in a doggie bag for a second meal the next day. You will also save money! This is called the "half and half" technique.

Ask for the senior menu.
These menus offer smaller portions at a reduced "ticket" price.

Forget what mom told you.
Never clean your plate. Restaurant portions are often two to four times bigger than your daily dietary needs.

Get your just desserts.
The new "hits" in the dessert department are low-calorie sorbet and fresh fruit. Share a dessert.

Fortifying Foods

Here is a list of AGE-less longevity foods sure to please your palate:

Whole grain bread: Beyond its terrific taste, each slice of whole-grain bread packs at least 3 grams of dietary fiber. And fiber fills you UP but doesn't fill you OUT. If you've been diagnosed with wheat intolerance, however, try some gluten-free breads or oatmeal breads.

Beans: Bring on the beans! One of my favorite weekend lunches is three-bean salad. Beans are excellent sources of protein. And, kidney beans, lima beans, black beans, and black-eyed peas are full of fiber—averaging between 6 to 8 grams of fiber per half-cup serving.

Nuts: Go a little nutty. Munch some almonds, walnuts, pecans or cashews each day. Or sprinkle a salad with sunflower seeds. In moderation, nuts and seeds are wonderful sources of monounsaturated fats—a true heart protector.

Fish: Get hooked on fish. Fresh or fresh-frozen fish is easily caught. So, don't pass up a plate of broiled or poached salmon. tuna, perch or cod. These fish (skip the butter) are swimming with omega-3 fatty acids, substances proven to elevate HDL cholesterol (your "healthy" type of fat that I call your "oil of delay"). An elevated HDL helps ward off arterial vascular disease. Fish oils also benefit joint function.

Avocados: I'm an advocate of avocados. Yes, I'm aware that this fruit is high in calories and contains about 30 grams of fat. BUT, a few slices of avocado in a salad or a sandwich offers you a tasty source of oleic acid, a monounsaturated fat. Or, you can get the same "healthy" fat from olive oil.

Strawberries: These bright red gems contain high levels of antioxidants. In fact, strawberries are part of an all-star cast of antioxidants that work to neutralize free radicals. In every stage at every age of life, free radicals are the villains, nasty particles that damage cells and can lessen the immune response.

Bananas and oranges: In combination, or as "solo acts," these fruits are touted to be loaded with blood-pressure-lowering potassium and vitamin C. They also boost your body's level of an enzyme that scientists suspect helps remove plaque from arterial walls. More good news about bananas: they also contain magnesium, necessary for bone strength and heart health.

Spinach and kale: Popeye would be proud to learn that these dark leafy greens are loaded with vitamin C and vitamin K—a lesser-known but vital vitamin that helps at least 12 proteins that assist blood cells, arteries and brain cells. These dark greens also contain lutein, an antioxidant that absorbs free radicals AND lessens the chance of developing cataracts. In fact, the Nurses' Health Study from Harvard reported that participants who ate spinach and kale regularly enjoyed up to 40 percent fewer cataract surgeries. Seeing IS believing! And kale is a super source of calcium.

Carrots: As Bugs Bunny would say, what's up, doc? Well, as a physician, I can tell you that carrots are considered cancer fighters. These orange veggies (as well as squash and pumpkin) contain chemicals that may inhibit tumor growth.

Tomatoes: Mama mia! I love tomatoes! Serve them to me sliced on sandwiches or simmering in a pasta sauce. Tomatoes contain lycopene, a potent antioxidant that may reduce the risk of prostate and lung cancers.

Grapes: Treat yourself to GRAPE expectations! Eating grapes and raisins, especially those with deeply colored skin, may protect you against heart disease and possibly prevent degenerative brain diseases such as Alzheimer's disease. Researchers at the University of Alabama at Birmingham's Center for the Study of Dietary Supplements in Botanicals report that polyphenols in soy suppress brain changes associated with Alzheimer's disease. Polyphenols in grapes deliver the same protection.

Red wine: Here is where I bend from The "LIQUIDATION Diet." Drinking two or three glasses of red wine a week is good for your digestion, temperament, and your heart. I'll drink to that! In moderation, of course! Wine may drive you to drink, but NEVER drink and drive!

Blueberries: Why not consider these baby blues for dessert instead of a thick slab of butterscotch cream pie? This very versatile berry can be added to cereals, salads, pancakes, muffins, smoothies, yogurt, sauces, chutney, and dessert toppings. One cup only contains 80 calories and ZERO grams of fat. Among 40 fruits and vegetables, blueberries rank number 1 in antioxidant activity. That's what researchers discovered after conducting a U.S. Department of Agriculture-sponsored study at the Human Nutrition Center on Aging at Tufts University in North Grafton, Massachusetts. Blueberries have been shown to improve balance, coordination, and memory. Wow! I want my thrill—on Blueberry Hill!

More Food-Friendly Facts

Here are a few more thoughts on how foods can keep you feeling WELLderly with some terrific recent "takes" on healthy headliners.

A call out to all coffee drinkers: In a long-term study of 8,004 Japanese-American men ages 45 to 68, experts concluded that moderate coffee drinkers have lower incidence of Parkinson Disease than peers who do not drink much or any coffee. Incidences of the disease ranged from 10.4 per 10,000 person-years in men who drank no coffee to 1.9 in men who drank at least 28 ounces per day. The study appeared in the *Journal of the American Medical Association.*

Today, when the "elite meet to eat," red meat is often used as condiment (as in Oriental cooking) to vegetables—seldom as the "main feature" on your plate. When eating out, select lean cuts of red meat or substitute beef with fowl or lean pork. Remember, fish is always a healthy winner.

Say "no thanks" as much as possible to foods containing saturated fats. Stay away from margarines and hydrogenated shortenings when preparing foods at home and when buying prepared foods such as snacks, bakery products, and candy. Check the label.

Don't forget to FAKE IT! You can liberally use no-fat "fake" butter, cheese, sour cream, mayonnaise and "no yolk" egg substitutes or egg whites. Fat-free hotdogs and fat-free sandwich meats are easy to find. Tofu, a soy product that is high in protein and low in fat, is also readily available. And, to satisfy that sweet tooth, there are fat-free candies—even fat-free chocolate!

Keep asking for the healthier choices. After all, demand and supply is the American way. Help drive the consumer market toward more products that are low in fat and do your part to help us all become more WELLderly.

Enlist Helpful Herbs

Fight aging the natural way by making sure nature's "green pharmacy"—medicinal herbs—are included in your daily script. Many of the mightiest of herbs are culinary delights—terrific to the taste! Work with your holistic-minded practitioner on which herbs in which forms work best for you.

To get you motivated, allow me to introduce my HERBAL HEADLINERS:

Garlic *(Allium sativum):* This "bulb of long life" lowers cholesterol, lowers blood pressure, and reduces the chance of blood clots developing. Garlic also acts like a nifty germ fighter because it is a natural antimicrobial. So, toss a few cloves of garlic into your pasta sauces, soups, or stir-fried vegetables. Onions, to a lesser degree, offer many of the same great traits as garlic.

Green tea: After dinner, I skip a cup of coffee and treat myself to a cup of green tea instead. With each sip, I'm happy knowing that this drink contains polyphenols and catechins, compounds that protect my heart by lowering cholesterol. They also act as powerful antioxidants and are believed to be part of the cancer-fighting army.

Saw Palmetto *(Serenoa repens):* Gentlemen, this well-studied herb can actually help shrink enlarged protstates and restore normal urine flow. Even better, take it to PREVENT any prostate problems.

Black Cohosh *(Cimicifuga racemosa):* Ladies, this well-studied herb has received RAVE reviews for decades in Europe as a natural way to reduce hot flashes and mood swings associated with menopause.

Ginkgo *(Ginkgo biloba):* Good news for folks with fuzzy memories. Among herbs, ginkgo tops the list as a memory booster. Its active compounds improve blood flow and provide oxygen to the brain to help you think more clearly. Ginkgo also reduces anxiety, lowers blood pressure, and relieves tension headaches and tinnitus (ringing in the ears).

I know what you're about to say: *If ginkgo is so good for my memory, how can I remember to take it?* The best time to take gingko is in the morning so that it can work all day long. To remember to take ginkgo, store the ginkgo bottle next to a drinking glass on the kitchen counter, next to a glass on the bathroom sink, or with your car keys. In no time, you'll be starting a healthy habit—and improving your memory. Be patient. It takes six to eight weeks of continual ginkgo usage before you'll notice any benefits.

Caution on Garlic and Gingko

Consult your physician before eating garlic or taking gingko if you are taking anticoagulant medicine to thin your blood or preparing for surgery. As a good rule, always make your physician aware of the herbs and supplements you take.

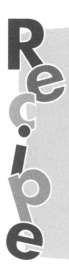

Memory-Boosting Tea

The next time you're searching for some clear thoughts, try this brain-aid tea:

1 teaspoon dried peppermint leaves
½ teaspoon dried ginkgo leaves
½ teaspoon dried rosemary leaves
1 teaspoon honey (optional)

In a small container, mix the herbs. Scoop 1 teaspoon of herbal mix into a cup of boiling water. Cover and let steep for about 10 minutes.

Dr. Dale's Dandy Tip

Please visit the National Institute on Health's Office of Dietary Supplements online (www.ods.od.nih.gov) to educate yourself about ingredients in supplements. There are many false and misleading sources of health information, especially on the Internet. When surfing the net, seek advice from web sites ending with .gov or .org and always consult your health care practitioner.

Sensational Supplements

Simply popping a pill, even a multi-vitamin, is no guarantee that you will stay fit—or even learn to fiddle! But seriously, HOLISTIC physicians are now firm believers in a once or twice daily multi-vitamin-mineral-supplement regiment. Supplements should not be substitutes for a good diet, but they are fill-ins that are needed when some of the nutritional "chorus" or supporting cast may be missing.

Please get into the habit of taking a multi-vitamin/mineral each day. Scientists at the Jean Mayer USDA Human Nutrition Research Center on Aging at Tufts University in Boston conducted an eight-week clinical trial with 80 healthy men and women with an average age of 67. The trial indicated that seniors who take multivitamin/mineral supplements each day had improvements in the blood levels of most nutrients—key to reducing the chance of chronic diseases. The supplement included 13 vitamins and 14 minerals, most at 100 percent of the daily value.

AGEless Wisdom

Winning smiles makes winners of us all.

Nutritional studies now suggest that mineral deficiencies or imbalances are likely contributing to many health disorders. Clearly all body systems and functions depend on basic minerals. But, modern farming, inadequate diets, medications and faulty gut absorption could lead to mineral deficits. Therefore, the wisdom of modest, mineral supplementation has become recognized by many nutritionists and health care providers. The benefit of minierals in an oral, electrolyte solution appears to be especially promising.

> ### AGEless Wisdom
> It doesn't hurt to laugh.

In reading the label, make sure that a multi-vitamin/mineral product contains selenium. This trace mineral often gets overshadowed by the more heralded antioxidants: vitamins A, C, and E. Win the game of life with these antioxidant ACES. ACES is a powerful acronym for good health.

Selenium and the antioxidants activate body enzymes that protect cells against free-radical molecules. Selenium also works in tandem with vitamin E, promoting normal cell growth and development. Selenium may:

- Relieve arthritic pain and discomfort
- Protect against cardiovascular disease, strokes, and heart attacks
- Remove unsightly age spots when rubbed on hands
- Reduce high blood pressure
- Help cure certain types of cancers (prostate, colon, and lung)

A recent study published in the *Journal of the National Cancer Institute* reported that men who ate 160 micrograms of selenium daily cut their risk of prostate cancer by about 65 percent compared with men who ingested less than 85 micrograms of selenium per day. Another study published in the *Journal of the American Medical Association* showed that taking daily supplements of 200 micrograms of selenium could reduce the risk of prostate, colon, and lung cancers by up to 63 percent.

Aching joints, sore muscles and arthritis can make us feel OLDER. Relief can be found by partnering up chondroitin sulfate with glucosamine. Preliminary studies suggest that this combination can ease the aches and limited mobility associated with arthritis—minus any serious side effect. My patients with osteoarthritis also report that these supplements work for them.

Bedtime Booster—Ta Tums!

Before you turn off the house lights—don't drink a glass of warm milk. Skip that bowl of ice cream. Milk and ice cream can often thicken mucus secretions that aggravate congestion, cough and hoarseness. Instead, I urge you to take Tums, Rolaids or Titralac before you head for bed. These stomach acid neutralizers will reduce stomach acids and "keep your nose clean" and control nighttime coughs. These calcium carbonate chewables help preserve the healthy "youthful" voice and improve breathing at night. Congestion of the head, throat and lungs are typically caused by:
Bacteria, Viruses, Smoking, Allergies
AND—GERD (gastro-esophageal reflux disorder)

If you wonder why you cough more when you lie down or why your sinuses fill up at night or why you're hoarse upon awakening, the "villain" is stomach acid vapors. These gaseous fumes back up the esophagus when you are lying down and they irritate the mucosa of your nose, throat, and lungs.

That's where Tums, Rolaids, Titralac or an equivalent can come to your aid. I recommend that you eat three or four of these chewables at bedtime to neutralize your stomach acids. Your stomach will be happy, your sinuses and your lungs will be glad and your bones will be ecstatic with these bone-preserving calcium treats.

And finally, if grandma was here to tuck you in, she would give you a warm hug and a hot brandy with water and honey to sip. If you are not averse to sipping this small amount of alcohol, you will discover that brandy can thin respiratory secretions, warm the body, and invite sound sleep. Then grandma would whisper, "You are loved," tuck you in, turn off the house lights and hum, "Tomorrow is the opening of another show!"

Good night! You're getting your ACT together WELL!

And whisper:
BRAVO!
SHHHH!

AGEless Wisdom

Health and Happiness are laughing matters.

Ageless Ally

Barbara Huebner

Barbara Huebner is living proof that life does get better with age. She didn't learn to downhill ski until age 40. She took up yoga at age 61. And, although she has golfed since age 12, she didn't sink her first hole-in-one until age 48.

At the young age of 71, Barbara happily reports that she has notched not one, but FOUR holes-in-one, with the latest one occurring shortly after her 70th birthday. She swung her 6-iron and watched the ball sail 115 yards before plopping down on the green and making a straight path to the flag and in the hole on a course in Mission Viejo, California.

"My first hole-in-one at age 48 was a terrible shot—form-wise," laughs Barbara, a retired school teacher who now volunteers to teach English to adults from foreign countries. "It bumped along on the fairway and ran up onto the green and into the hole. But, my fourth hole-in-one was so beautiful. The tee shot floated up in the air, landed softly on the green and right into the cup."

Barbara symbolizes the payoffs of being persistent—and positive. Playing golf and performing yoga gives her more energy and offers her a chance to spend quality time with family and friends.

"I've always had a youthful outlook and never felt mature," she says. "I've never felt more than about age 25."

She pauses and then adds: "A lot of people my age seem to look at life as having only a limited number of years left. They seem to worry that they won't have enough time to do this or do that. As for me, I wake up every day feeling great. If you stay active and do things for others, you'll feel less sorry for yourself and truly enjoy life."

ACT 4

Play Out A
DRAMATIC HIT
Start a HAPPY-demic!

In order to ACT well, you must first acknowledge and discard your "old, negative parts." Because how you think, how you react to situations, how you move, sit and stand and the words you select to say all play roles in your overall health. For a more exciting new WELLderly role you will want to reset the stage and put a newer, more fun act together. And then play it out in the new State Theater of Everyday Life.

Recent scientific findings reinforce the long-standing observation that the human body, when given the opportunity, seems to opt for optimism over pessimism. Renowned psychologist and clinical researcher Martin Seligman has studied optimists and pessimists for more than 25 years. His groundbreaking book, *Learned Optimism: How To Change Your Mind and Your Life*, defines pessimists as people who believe that bad events undermine everything and these events are their fault. Conversely, optimists, according to Dr. Seligman, view defeats as temporary setbacks or challenges.

"People are about as happy as they make up their minds to be."
ABRAHAM LINCOLN

We all need—AND DESERVE—a positive attitude tune-UP, especially when you consider the price that pessimists pay. Here are some concrete reasons to TRANCE-form those frowns into smiles and those woe-is-me thoughts into WOW-is-me thoughts and actions:

- The more optimistic a person is at age 20, the healthier he or she will likely be at 60.
- Pessimists are more likely to develop cancer than optimists.
- Pessimists with heart disease tend to die before optimists with heart woes.

We can't and should not laugh everything off and always peer through rose-colored glasses, BUT we will feel better if we do just that. Remember feelings are chemistry and the A.C.T. approach is that **AC**Tions and **T**houghts change our "**C**hemistry." Yes, act happy—BE happy. And the more one rehearses the part the more it becomes "real." And real happy people on average live longer—really!

A good "hearty" laugh seems to be good for your heart. People with heart disease were 40 percent LESS likely to laugh in humorous situations than folks with healthy hearts, based on a study conducted by researchers at the Center for Preventative Cardiology at the University of Maryland.

> **AGEless Wisdom**
>
> LIGHTEN UP and the world is brighter and more beautiful.

Optimistic OR pessimistic attitudes can be traced to the brain's emotion-generating limbic system and its thought-generating cerebral cortex. Even "born pessimists" have the capacity to convert to optimism. We can all change our tune and have new UPbeat music play and be recorded in the chambers of our heart.

In the words of General Douglas MacArthur:

> *"You are as young as your faith, as old as your doubt;*
> *as young as your self-confidence, as old as your fear;*
> *as young as your hope, as old as your despair. In the*
> *central place of your heart, there is a recording cham-*
> *ber; so long as it receives messages of beauty, hope,*
> *cheer, and courage, so long you are young."*

I salute the late great general for such inspiring words!

Nobody grows old by merely living a specific number of years. People grow old only by abandoning their ideals. Years may wrinkle the skin, but to give up one's interests and passions will wrinkle the soul. Worry, doubt, anxiety, fear and despair can rob one of the joy of life—if you let this negative chemistry steal your show.

Even "bad hair days" can make our self-esteem go awry, according to a Yale University study conducted by psychology researchers. On those days, people unable to "tame their locks" feel less smart, less capable, less sociable and more embarrassed. So, in reality, all those who make us look better are health care providers. They help us feel better.

> **AGEless Wisdom**
>
> "The best way to make your audience laugh is to start laughing yourself."
>
> Oliver Goldsmith

The Power of WE in WEllness

Remember the importance of surrounding yourself with happy, healthy friends and family. We can't ACT the happy role alone. Two or more are needed if we hope to play off someone else's chemistry. There is only one letter, an "I" in I-llness, but two, a powerful "WE" in WE-llness.

One of the most miraculous re-IN-ACTments of medical improvement was enjoyed by my patient, Gertie. She first started coming to me for care several years ago. Whenever she walked on the "clinic stage" it was obvious she was in the "I" role. She had only inward, "me" thoughts. And the body followed the thoughts. Her tired, weak, aching body was tucked IN, Down and Backwards. Her complaint: "I'm sick and tired of being all IN." She was in the posture, thoughts and chemistry that actors on stage assume to play the "sad" part. The same body posture and thoughts that get actors into the "chemistry" of being in old, tired, defeated, dejected, weak and sick roles. All these parts look the same. They all have the same appearance of a turning IN, a sinking, shrinking DOWN and a falling BACKWARDS. Just the opposite of the UP, OUT and FORWARD position of the happy part.

On one of Gertie's frequent office visits, I said, "Gertie, please take this piece of paper and pen. Write down these letters:

LLNESS

At this point in her life, her aches and pains were taking Center Stage.

"Gertie, are you sick and tired of being all IN?"

In her tucked-in, weakened, and sinking posture she whispered with a tear in her eye: "Yes."

"Okay, Gertie, then write the letter, "I" in front of the letters,

I LLNESS

My actress patient featured in ACT 1 taught me that the happy part was played UP, OUT and FORWARD. I wanted to share this with Gertie. I wanted to help Gertie learn that by playing a new part of an UPbeat happy person and by connecting with the outside world she would be able to come OUT of her "old" painful part. If she would move FORWARD, her being had the potential of connecting with the UP, OUT and FORWARD chemistry that a stage performer uses to TRANCE-act and INstall a feel-good chemistry.

"Gertie, if you would try this stage method you may come out of some of your self-centered misery. You just might be able to reconnect, to become a part of rather than apart from your friends and family—you could write new letters in front of LLNESS.

"Gertie–try WE!"

"For you, Dr. Anderson, anything—even if it's silly—is worth my try."

She then boldly put the letters "WE" in front of LLNESS. She looked at the two word possibilities and whispered, "I-LLNESS" and, almost with a shout and a chuckle she blurted, "WE-LLNESS" Her eyes sparkled and a rare smile illuminated her face.

I smugly boasted to myself, "by Jove, she's got it!"

WE
LLNESS
I

And she DID get it, she DID begin to move UP, OUT and FORWARD, away from her aches and pains.

And almost everyone can, to a degree, at least improve their medical and emotional condition. Better the "chemistry" of how they feel. And some (hopefully you) like Gertie will have profound improvement. (See Appendix—CRIB Sheet—Fun, Happy, Healthy ACT UP, OUT and FORWARD.) (Gertie stars again in ACT 5.)

ACTitude Adjustment

You can start this instant by getting rid of old nagging, negatives words from the vocabulary and ACTitude. Boot out these no-good negative phrases:

> I have nothing to look forward to.
> I'm TOO old to do it.
> I'm just wearing out.
> I'm not as young as I used to be.
> Old folks get no respect. We're in the way.
> It has ALWAYS been that way.
> I can't stand it!
> At least I've got my memories.

Give your attitude an adjustment by accentuating the positive and look for more UPbeat and positive words. Let's rephrase and praise new, welcoming thoughts such as:

> Wow! What a refreshingly new way to attack this problem.
> I can become childlike without becoming childish.
> It's about time we tried something new.
> I'm up for new challenges!
> A little pain can be expected, and it's better than no pain at all.
> I'm happy and lucky to be alive.
> Let's work together to solve this problem.
> Nothing like a good new challenge to make life interesting.
> We don't have to win to have fun playing the game of life.
> Read any good books, seen any good movies lately?
> Let's get together and share a few chuckles.
> Ha! We laughed so hard I forgot my pains.

By speaking in a positive way and connecting with the eyes, you come across as more receptive and open to others. This makes everyone more comfortable and it allows you to be more creative and credible.

New for "OLD" Words

There are a few more word replacements I'd like you to consider. Why say "old" when "vintage" sounds so much better? Why say, "antique" when you can say "classic?" When I speak to "age-advantaged" peer groups, I tell my audiences to shun the script of becoming old or an antique but to proudly become a *VINTAGE CLASSIC*. And why be the "senior citizen" when you can be a VP (Vintage Person)!

And you should and can...

> ## Knock the "EL" out of __derly and become WELLderly!

Come on! Live it UP, OUT and FORWARD.

Pep Up Your Posture

Stand UP for the role you want to play. Now that we've got you talking the talk, we need to convince you that you must perfect the moves and walk the walk of youthful happiness to play OUT your part WELL.

When it comes to proper sitting and standing postures, our dear moms were certainly NO SLOUCHES! No sir! Moms knew best—and had a healthy point—each time they would "nag" us as children to stand up or sit up straight with shoulders back. We should have listened. Now, besides making us look better and younger, we understand why slouches suffer from decreased lung capacity, poor muscle tone and chronic pains. Slouches feel achy.

Free yourself from these pains by being UP, OUT and FORWARD! It's not to late to make improvements.

Good posture helps you avoid appearing like a LOM (Little Old Man) or LOL (Little Old Lady)—the IN, DOWN and BACK-WARD folks that look older than their years. Quite often, the key culprits to many aches and pains—and a downtrodden mood—can be these poor slouched sitting and standing postures. Over years, poor body position can lead to rounded lower backs, humped upper back, rolled shoulders and the forward-jutting of the chin along with a host of woes: back pain, neck aches, headaches and breathing difficulty.

In this "Internet Age," more folks are seated in front of a computer monitor and tap, tap, tapping on a keyboard. Time can ZIP by and as you move from one web site to the next or read an ava-lanche of emails, guess what tends to happen to your posture?

Perhaps without even realizing it, you l-e-a-n your head closer to the screen. Your shoulders round forward to accommodate your typing fingers. Your back curves like the letter, C. Your head, which weighs about the same as a 15-pound bowling ball, feels heavier when you slouch because of the tight pull on your upper posterior neck and back muscles. The results? The obvious, the inevitable happens—backache, headache and neck ache. And the LOL, LOM appearance.

Let's get those neck, shoulder, and back muscles feeling fit, and if not fabulous, at least feeling better again. Get out of your slump! Try these pain-free posture pointers for standing and sitting:

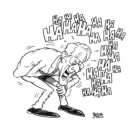

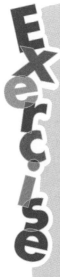

Stand Tall

Step 1. Keep your ears over your shoulders. Do NOT lean your head forward.

Step 2. Hold your head high and keep your chin parallel to the ground.

Step 3. Align your ear with your rear and the shoulders over your hips. Don't pull your shoulders way back, just keep them slightly back and relaxed.

Step 4. Lift your breastbone and maintain a little inward curve at your lower back. Keep your knees unlocked.

Now that I have you standing tall, it's time to get you "sitting tall."

Sit Tall

Step 1. Keep both feet flat on the floor.

Step 2. Sit up straight keeping the ear, the rear and the shoulder aligned. Some support for the low back will help maintain a slight inward curve of the lumbar spine.

Step 3. Make sure your head is sitting straight above the shoulders. Re-training your sitting posture isn't that hard. You just need to be diligent.

Remind yourself to arch your lower back whenever you sit. In time, your "internal computer" will "run the program" automatically and will make sure that you are sitting or standing in a healthful posture. The new chemistry will become a comfortable habit. It will begin to feel REAL.

Change for the better takes time—sometimes months—but the eventual difference can be AMAZING! Over time, I've seen 70-year-old VPs improve their posture and lessen their pain significantly by following these easy steps. If you need a little extra help, check ACT 6 for some great posture exercises for you to practice.

Slip Into A Smile

One of the most important "costumes" you can put on for good health is a smile. Your day goes the way the corners of your mouth go. When the corners of your mouth are UP, you're UP also. It is far more important what you wear ear to ear and year to year than what you wear from head to toe. By costuming your face in this way, you get more "smileage" out of life.

When you look at picture proofs and you select the ones to reprint, do you pick the smiling pictures? Of course! Why? Do you feel better about these pictures?

As we discussed in ACT 1, feelings are chemistry and chemistry is feelings, so your picture choices are proof positive that a smile changes your chemistry.

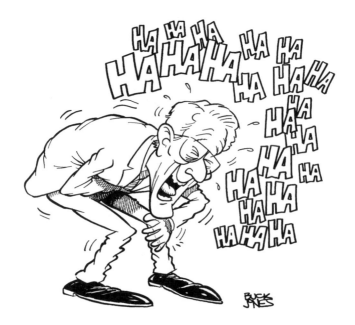

SPREAD A HAPPY-DEMIC

Smiles are priceless and contagious.
Smiling is infectious.
You catch it like the flu.

When someone smiled at me today,
I started smiling too.
I passed around the corner
and others saw my grin.

When they smiled, I realized
I'd passed it on to them.
I thought about that smile,
then I realized its worth.

A single smile, just like mine
could travel 'round the world.

So, if you feel a smile begin,
don't leave it undetected.

Let's start a HAPPYdemic quick,
and get the world infected!
—Unknown

Fill and Refill This Prescription

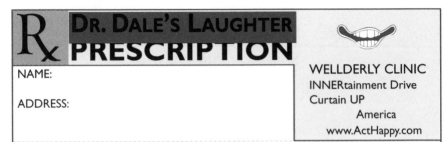

DR. DALE'S LAUGHTER PRESCRIPTION

NAME:

ADDRESS:

WELLDERLY CLINIC
INNERtainment Drive
Curtain UP
America
www.ActHappy.com

In front of mirror
Belly Laugh
15 seconds, 2x/Day

Unleash your feel-fabulous endorphins and relax tense muscles by following the "doctor's orders." Live it UP. Lighten UP and Laugh it OFF!

For many patients who need to "open UP," I actually take out my prescription pad and fill out a "laughter prescription." I scribble down these words: "In front of the mirror, belly laugh for 15 seconds, two times a day."

This Laughter Rx has been prescribed to my audiences around the world. Whether in Asia, Australia, Africa, Europe or North America, this universal language of laughter is the same. And it is not only universally spoken, but also universally understood. The prescription helps those in any culture "start UP" their "Laugh motors." When a group takes the Rx they laugh TOGETHER. The group bonds with each other. And good feelings are shared.

When you take this Dr. Dale's Laughter Rx, I'm not suggesting you do just any ordinary laugh. What we're after here is an all-out, bellowing, no-holds-barred, from-the-belly laugh. Not just a giggle or a little twitter but a body-flailing, arms-flinging, belly-holding, thigh-slapping, knee-buckling guffaw! My friend Merrilyn Belgum, Minnesota's 77-year-old "Queen Mother of Comedy" advises, "It's better to have laughed and leaked than never to have laughed at all."

Laughter can give you a good workout. One solid minute of laughter is worth about 40 minutes of deep relaxation and 100 laughs are equal to the same calories burned in a 10-minute jog, according to research by renowned physician William Fry, M.D.

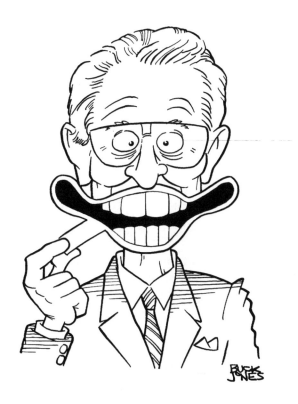

Here are the nine steps to achieving healing laughter

1. Stand in front of a mirror and "costume" your face. Mirrors are good tools for promoting laughter because they help "reflect" and "reframe" your new character. Just smile at yourself. Share a smile with yourself. Improve your face value. Think, "The me I see is the me I'll be!"

2. Widen your smile. Open your mouth enough to show a few teeth. Get your cheeks into the act and if you've got dimples, let 'em dance with delight.

3. Crinkle your eyes. This small act will start the release of "endorphins," according to some studies. After all, "a crinkle adds a twinkle" to your eyes. When people laugh, you can see it in their eyes. They light UP!

4. Lift your forehead. Raise the eyebrows and wiggle them UP and down. Show more teeth—open the mouth a bit—grin and bare those molars!

5. Add sound. Start with a few ha ha's. Try to generate these sounds from your diaphragm instead of your throat. Your aim is to achieve a "gut" laugh. Pretend you're Santa and you're laughing from the belly. Place your hands on your lower ribs and move the ha-ho-hee motion toward that area.

6. Pump up the laugh volume. Release a string of ha-ha-ha's. Each time, laugh a little bit louder and faster.

7. Once you've got your laughter engine hitting all cylinders, you need to engage the rest of your body. As you laugh, stand up tall, propel your head and shoulders upward and arch your back. At the same time, instruct your body to loosen up and lighten up.

8. Throw your arms UP, OUT and FORWARD. Raise your hands high over your head. Wiggle your fingers and gesture to the reflection in the mirror.

9. Now for the grand finale. Bring your hands down and slap your knees or thighs. Bend up and down at the waist. Hop UP and dance and turn on the legs. Jingle, jangle, gyrate—anything—everything! Keep laughing out loud the whole time. Pull all these steps together so you are PERFORMING in one free-flowing motion.

Back to Dr. Dale's Laughter Rx

A Minnesota "Laugh Out"

At first "blush" an occasional patient can't seem to crank out those chuckles. For those who are initially laugh-challenged, here's another option. Practice relocating the throat Ha-Ha's to the diaphragm where REAL laughter truly belongs. To teach audiences how to do this "belly laugh" I share the "Minnesota Cold Car Start" exercise.

Try this: pretend you're in Minnesota. It's 30 degrees below zero. It's morning and you are about to start a cold car. Imagine you have a cold key in your cold hand. You insert it into the ignition and you turn the key once and the car just moans a weak, one A-haa and then silence. Then with frosted breath, you say, "Please car, start UP, warm UP, become a hum-a-dinger." Once more, you turn the ignition and get A-haa, ha-h. And nothing more.

On the third try, you pray that it's going to catch, you visualize it as a laughing engine that is going to purr. And it does!

A-ha, ha, ha HA-HA-HA-HA!!! As you pretend to have a similar engine at the level of the diaphragm, can you feel that in the gut? It feels so good. Now, you can't stop. Put your hands on your belly and you can feel this full-throttle, from-the-diaphragm laughter.

Whatever you do, don't choke! Keep practicing and you'll get your laughter motor running on all cylinders in no time. And you'll be a true hum-a-dinger!

Each time you finish your glorious guffaws, take a few minutes to analyze the effects of your ACT. Do you notice any changes in your thinking, your chemistry, and your mood? Of course! You experience and now understand that laughter creates and releases a flood of neuropeptides. Proof positive that feeling good IS a laughing matter!

Some people might say, "I can't do this at home or at work. If I do this laughter prescription, they will laugh at me."

That's true. At first they will laugh AT and then they will laugh WITH. Because what is more spreading, more catching, more infectious than laughter? There is no easier way to start a HAPPY-demic than to be around people who are laughing. We gravitate to laughter; we are pulled to the people who we can share laughter with.

Bu$ine$$

And "healthy" businesses can bank on laughter, too. Happy employees are more creative and productive. They have far fewer sick days. And customers come back to businesses where they experience an UPbeat happy chemistry. Business can "bank on IT." And IT is the chemistry of prosperous happiness.

Connect with Laugher—Start A Laughter Group

You read right. My physician friend, Madan Kataria of Bombay (Mumbai) India is a doctor that has become a renowned proponent of unconditional laughter. He has spurred the formation of Laughter Clubs all over the globe. His groups all operate on the simple premise that unconditional, FAKED laughter generates happiness and health. Dr. Kataria's happy laughter yoga exercises are like organized cheers.

When I visited Dr. Kataria in Bombay several years ago I participated in a number of these Indian Laughter Clubs that gathered in city parks. I was cheered on by a designated "laugh-leader." With my new Indian friends I was able to celebrate again the reality that laughter makes a happy environment and should be the "glue" that helps hold a peaceful world together.

Wisdom says, "I love those with whom I laugh."

For Dr. Kataria, laughter is a mantra—the same staged technique that METHOD Actors have always practiced to turn ON for an UPbeat performance. When we met in India; we excitedly shared our enthusiasm about his Laughter Club Movement and the ACT NOW Project and Foundation.

I was able to share the Laughter Rx and J'ARMing with his groups, and later, when he and his wife Madhuri visited Minnesota, he regaled my hospital staff and several gatherings at my home with his enthusiastic zeal.

Dr. Kataria's book, *LAUGH for No Reason* and web site are listed in the appendix. As are the web sites for Joel Goodman's Humor Project, The World Laughter Tour, and the Association of Applied and Therapeutic Humor.

Of course, you are always invited to share your UPlifting thoughts and talents by visiting www.ActHappy.com, the web site for the ACT NOW Project and the ACT NOW Foundation.

If you are a budding poet or word-right, it's time to play it UP and create UP and share UP and serve UP some of your UP ideas to cheer UP others—an UP poem, UP affirmation, UP short saying or UP paragraph using as many UP phrases as possible. A collection of these **"UP" Rights** that are suitable for grade school children is being worked UP for future publication. And your contribution, if selected and original, would be credited to you. Make UP something now and enjoy being written UP.

If you're UP to it, check UP on all the "clean" UP phrases in the appendix.

Think UP or Dream UP an UPlifting message that will help others live it UP!

As an affirmation example:

It's UP to me!
Today I'll measure UP!
I'll get UP, cheered UP and
will keep UP showing UP, UP!
I'll store UP, add UP, save UP and
Finish UP this day "high" on life.
Today, I will live IT UP!
It's UP to me!
Curtain UP!
You're ON!
BRAVO!

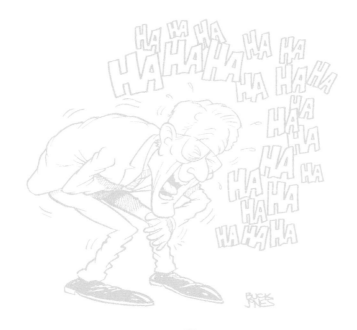

Ageless Ally

Meet Maryann "Annie" Glasgow, a very youthful 66-year-old psychotherapist and a big birthday booster in St. Paul, Minnesota. She is never without positive energy, a quick smile, and a full, infectious laugh.

Like many of us, she's endured her share of life's challenges and traumas. Her husband of 25 years died of a heart attack and one of her sons suffered a chronic disabling injury from an automobile accident. She had every right to retreat, to be negative.

"That would be the easy way out, but I've learned to rebuild, to reinvent myself, to help others live life with enthusiasm," she says.

As a psychotherapist—and occasional professional clown—Annie gently restores the vibrancy of LIFE in children who had been abused, working professionals burned out by too many deadlines, and retirees dueling depression.

Annie says it is important to have role models in your life, fine folks who motivate and inspire you. One of Annie's guiding lights is the feisty, spirited Isabella Cannon, who ran and won the mayoral election in Raleigh, North Carolina when she was in her seventies. That was 25 YEARS ago! Last year, Isabella wowed an audience as the commencement speaker for a college in North Carolina at age 96.

"Don't forget to thank your role models," says Annie. "Isabella has a collection of angel figurines, and I recently found a porcelain angel statue holding the world in her hands. I immediately thought of Isabella and sent it with a note thanking her for being my guardian angel."

Annie lives by the motto: "Add years to your life and life to your years!"

And, demonstrating her quick wit, she adds with a twinkle in her eye: "Age is important only if you are a cheese."

She's absolutely right.

Maryann "Annie" Glasgow

ACT

The
SUPPORTING CAST
Team UP WE–ll

Great actors are quick to acknowledge their supporting casts. They know their starring roles would not be as illuminating if it were not for actors playing minor roles and all the folks behind the scenes.

As an actor on the stage of life, you, too, need to take the time to shine the spotlight on the Three Ps: people, pets, and plants… plus more!

Great mates RATE in my book! Same goes for best friends. The secret to happy marriages, relationships and terrific friendships includes the ability to be playful and childlike.

I suggest that you "set the stage and script" for specific times to connect with others, and not just your physician. Treat these times as you would a business appointment or a trip to your beautician or barber. Keep a calendar and block out times when you plan to see friends, or enjoy a quiet, relaxed dinner with your partner, or visit your children or grandchildren.

Recently, I enjoyed an outing with my 8-year-old grandson, Ethan. I blocked out the morning for us to go to the Minnesota

"If you can make it better, you can laugh at it."
ERMA BOMBECK

Science Museum to visit the "Oh, Gross" special exhibit on gross body functions. A bit of grandfather/grandson, man-to-man bonding. The exhibits were the subject of my daily work and the brunt of my grandson's jokes. We both joked; we both laughed. And we now share a happy "gross" memory. The point is to take time with your grandchild or young people for the sheer "health" of it—for all of you!

The Universal Main Frame

Finally, set aside times for your spiritual practice, whatever that is. Regular church/synagogue/mosque attendance, prayer, or meditation can increase your sense of being connected. The beneficial power of prayer has proven itself over and over again.

Spiritually, all religions use their favorite "software" to access the CREATOR. But once one connects through the www (world wide web) of understanding we discover that the "Source," The Hard Drive, The Main Frame is the same for all earthlings.

As a student at Carleton College 50 years ago, I was planning to become a pastor. Until, that is, I enrolled in a course on Russian history. There I encountered Karl Marx's quote: "Religion is the opium of the people." That thought disturbed me a great deal. Sleepless nights. I gave up pre-seminary aspirations. Now, years later, understanding the new science of psychoneuroimmunology and endorphins—the morphine within—it is evident that Karl Marx was right. The chemistry of religion, of spirituality, of connecting to a "higher power" gives way to better health. Amen!

Cuddle Your Canine—Or Your Cat

Patients who are feeling blue are encouraged to get a "fur fix." If you're not allergic, adopt a dog or a cat—and watch the healing power of pets kick in with each tail wag or full-throttle purr.

The strongest optimism-producing sensation you possess is touch. You can elevate your mood by petting and cuddling with a dog or cat, creatures that give you unconditional love. And you can help your health, too. Even surrogate pets like teddy bears and stuffed animals have been shown to positively impact feelings— and consequently health.

AGEless Wisdom
Make Your Pleasures Habits.

Cats and canines are natural calmers. People with dogs by their sides had lower blood pressure and heart rates than folks "dog-less" in a study conducted by researchers at the University of Buffalo School of Medicine and Biomedical Sciences in New York. Mayo Clinic research has found that elderly people who have pet companions have a lower incidence of cancer. Pets are also heralded for their abilities to prevent, detect, speed recovery, and in some cases, cure a variety of maladies.

One study of people over 65 living alone who owned dogs showed they needed physicians 16 percent less than those who were dog-less. This is a difficult admission for any physician, that we can be replaced by a dog 16 percent of the time. I guess our practice, in part, has gone to the dogs!

And recently, it was a privilege to be spotlighted as an expert in a *Cat Fancy* magazine cover story that addressed 10 ways cats help folks soothe frayed nerves and relax snarled muscle knots. Cats—and dogs—are nature's underrated—and overlooked—form of Prozac. Our pets have the ability to raise our levels of serotonin, endorphins and other feel-good body chemicals.

Are you as curious as, say, a CAT to learn how your feline friend (and canine chum) can be your surprising health ally to fight stress? Here are 10 perks to sharing your life with a pet.

10 Ten perks to sharing your life with a pet

Pets:

1. **Act as natural yoga teachers.** They know the value of purposeful stretching to work muscle groups BEFORE vacating that warm spot on your bed.

2. **Know the therapeutic value of touch.** They aren't shy about asking for hugs. So seek out hugs and therapeutic massages from family and friends to unknot those muscle snarls on your neck, shoulders and back.

3. **Know the value of solitude.** Spending some time alone each day is vital to re-charge.

4. **Know the value of power napping.** Your dog and cat use these mini-naps throughout the day to recharge and revive. If you could take a 10-minute afternoon nap, you will be in talented company. Many creative people, including inventor Thomas Edison, were power nappers.

5. **Know the importance of eating right.** This applies more to cats than your in-the-garbage-can-again canine.

6. **Walk away from irritating scenes.** Who needs to be confronted constantly by stress-raising situations?

7. **Live in the present.** They don't get caught up in the "should haves" and "what ifs" way of thinking that only BREEDS guilt, stress, and worry.

8. **Are candid.** They ask for what they want—and if the answer is NO, they move on.

9. **Practice good hygiene.** Again, this applies more to never-have-a-bad-hair-day cats, not rolled-in-the-mud-again dogs. When you shower, shave and fix your hair, you feel better inside and out. You feel good, so you smile, a natural and healthy reaction.

10. **Are not materialistic.** In the desperate attempt to keep up with the Joneses, the toll can go beyond your wallet. You also feel stress and frustration.

Leaf It to Plants

Let's "branch out" a bit and speak of the power of petunias. And roses. And all of Mother Nature's beautiful botanicals. Sharing your life with plants CAN ease your stress, lower blood pressure, fend off headaches and speed your recovery after surgery.

We have yet to pinpoint precisely WHY plants improve people's health. But we can confirm that plants do release oxygen and moisture, two elements that create more of a comfy, cozy home. Plants purify the air and absorb pollutants and they can help mask noise and glare.

Officials at the American Horticultural Therapy Association shared with me a fascinating study. They compared the blood pressure levels of folks performing identical tasks. One group did these chores in a greenhouse surrounded by lush vegetation and the other group did these chores in a training center with nary a leaf in sight. The results: the greenhouse gang displayed significantly lower systolic and diastolic blood pressure than those in the plant-less work plant.

I attribute plants to helping one of my chronic pain patients, Gertie (same Gertie as Act 4), get a much-needed endorphin boost.

She lived alone in an apartment with only a television set for company. She had no close friends, no church or spiritual connection, and her family lived far away. The daily "news reports" were full of mayhem and disaster, aggravating the pains in her body.

"Gertie, why not consider adopting a dog or a cat? You know, to reconnect, to feel that special bond, to feel needed. To get some living in your life."

Unfortunately, she rented in a no-pet apartment complex.

"So, how about plants? Would you consider caring for a few plants? You'll find it an enjoyable hobby that gets you in touch with Mother Nature."

Gertie agreed and started with a few plants and a bottle of Miracle Grow. And miracles happened. She had quite an attentive "green thumb" and in no time she had an apartment adorned with healthy, vibrant plants. She said she was in "plant parenthood." She began sharing her plants with others in her apartment complex and started to cultivate many new friends. She gained the confidence to attend garden shows and garden lectures and her long-lost humor re-sprouted. She shared with me that at a recent flower show she met a "seedy" widowed farmer and she was trying to plant some "romantic ideas."

"No, I'm not trying to sow any 'wild oats'—yet!" she snickered.

Gertie was beginning to blossom. A late bloomer, you might say. But she had turned over a new leaf. She had become grounded in the endorphins and her aches and pains were being supplanted with happiness. Gertie proved to be a grand "plant parent" and her aches and pains were steadily weeded away. She brings plants into my office now. Once she brought in a flowering Amaryllis, planted it on my desk and said, "Dr. Anderson, this *bud's* for you!"

A simple living connection with plants was enough to transform Gertie from the achy role to an achieving role. What a re-leaf! And, what about that "seedy" farmer? Well, he is now MR. Gertie.

Added Pluses

A New "Hue"

Feel years younger by watching what you wear. When you want to relax, try slipping into a baby blue sweatshirt and sweat-pants. When you seek more energy, try pulling on a bright red sweater.

Scientists now acknowledge that colors "indeed" do color our moods. Cool colors like blues and greens help us relax after a tiring day. Warm colors like reds, oranges and yellows help us lighten up and get us going.

For the WELLderly, try wearing more youthful clothes. Look around and see what people 20 years younger than you are wearing. Don't wear outdated clothing like leisure suits or polyester pants. Not sure what to wear? Go to an airport or the theater and look what people in their 40s are wearing. Try to emulate that style. The fashions of the young middle-aged are always IN style—for every age.

And here's a fashion flash: what you wear that others can't see can influence your mood. One recent study on depressed people discovered that those individuals who put on flashy underwear became happier. Bravo for those heart-adorned boxers and those red panties! It's your inside joke—so wear it WELL! You will feel good "all under" all over.

The Good Sense Behind Scents

It's okay to be led by your nose.

Minnesota is home to the Mall of America, the mega place for shopping. This architectural wonder is so BIG that SEVEN Yankee Stadiums would fit inside. Why bring this up? Whenever I go there I am "led by the nose" to one of my favorite stores.

I find myself drifting toward a coffee shop with its warming, inviting aroma of freshly brewing coffee beans. My nose also picks up the nearby irresistible popcorn stand specializing in cinnamon caramel corn. I feel good here. Maybe it's the aromas of home that have triggered happy childhood memories.

I've learned through my holistic medicine training that I can behave with more calm in a traffic snarl if I spritz my car interior with lavender—a natural soothing smell. The science: lavender increases alpha brain rhythms, which are typical of a relaxed state. Jasmine triggers beta rhythms, associated with alertness.

A study of nearly 1,000 subjects conducted by the Smell and Taste Treatment and Research Foundation in Chicago discovered that VINTAGE people are more likely to spend more money at a store when they are exposed to natural scents, such as pine or hay.

This same group also discovered that gamblers spend nearly 53 percent more money at a Las Vegas casino when it was infused with a pleasant odor instead of being unscented. I guess that's what they mean by the "smell of money."

And speaking of money, you can re-decorate your home without taking out an equity loan. Scent your home with candles or aroma therapy oils. Evaluate which aromas elevate your mood. After all, your nose KNOWS!

What is YOUR aroma of happiness? Identify it and use it WELL. For some it may be vanilla; for others it could be peppermint. For me, sage is a happy smell and chocolate—OHHHH!

The Magic of Music

Music can promote health and serenity—a concept that has been known and embraced for centuries. About 2,500 years ago, philosopher Pythagoras was depicted on a papyrus singing and playing an instrument to purge negative emotions such as sorrow, worry and fear. This papyrus, according to Robert Ornstein and David Sobel, represents the oldest known medical document. And for you Greek mythology fans, let me remind you that the almighty Apollo was the god of both medicine AND music.

Although music has been with us since the very beginning, we are finally conducting some solid science behind its benefits. This science is called *cymatics*—the study of the effects of sounds and music on matter. And, believe me, people DO matter!

Music played for patients before, during and after surgery has resulted in reduced need for medication, less pain and anxiety, and faster recovery. Some obstetricians theorize that playing music for women during childbirth may reduce the length of labor and the pain.

And think of how much "nicer" it is when you're down in the mouth at your dentist's office and therapeutic music muffs the sound of the dreaded drill.

Music may also help you with your memory and concentration powers. The melodic notes can drown out irritating sounds and hone your focus so you can work more efficiently. And studies show that if you need to work on your memory skills, play classical music or instrumental jazz. If you want to sleep soundly, consider putting on classical or New Age music at bedtime. These types of music with a 60-beat-per-minute rhythm match, on average, your resting heart rate. Faster music and jazz are more likely to tune you UP and turn you ON. Jazz, marches, or "old fast dance favorites" will help you dial in to an UPbeat feeling. Live it UP each morning. Program UPbeat music to get UP, turn UP and start UP the INNER UPPERS. Wake UP, "high on life."

Yes, music, aromas, colors, plants, and pets can help "knock" the EL out of __DERLY and replace EL with WELL.

Be WELLderly!
BRAVO!

Ageless Allies

Roberta and John Mulliner

Roberta Mulliner, a highly efficient office manager, regarded her pending retirement with a bit of hesitation.

She was the definition of multi-tasker. She could juggle many jobs simultaneously and was the go-to person whenever co-workers at a major publishing company needed help.

When her company unexpectedly announced an early retirement buyout a few years before Roberta was ready to retire, it caught her uncharacteristically off-guard. She stopped and studied the offer's perks. She realized the best time to retire was NOW.

Years earlier, her husband, John, had retired from the truck driving business. The couple had settled into an uninspiring routine: she worked; he stayed home and fed the birds migrating through their eastern Pennsylvania backyard. Every Friday night they ate at the same nearby diner.

They had fallen deeply into a R-U-T.

"We needed to shake up our lives, so I suggested to John we move to Long Island," recalls Roberta. "It was one of the best decisions we've ever made."

Today, the Mulliners are marvelous WELLderly models. They've rediscovered life and their marriage is stronger than ever.

What's their ageless secret? They were willing to try something new together: kayaking. As long as the weather permits, they paddle the creeks and rivers threading through their peninsula town of Cutchogue, New York. They silently skim through the waters, basking in the warm sun, enjoying close-up views of fish and birds, and reveling in the joys of nature.

Chronologically, Roberta is 65, but she marks her life now by activities, not years. She volunteers at a hospice center and a hospital and loves touring local wineries with out-of-town guests.

"At my age, I'm comfortable with myself," she says. "Age brings you wisdom and the experience that goes along with it if you just let it."

ACT 6

IT'S SHOW TIME!
Take Center Stage

Taking on a new and improved, happy, WELLderly role takes time. You may feel awkward initially until the "new you"—the more positive you, the UPbeat you becomes an IN-ACTed habit. And, be tolerant of your family and friends. During your "transition," they may be perplexed by your changing personality and the new INproved chemistry you are creating.

The "old" you could have been somewhat of a grouch in the morning and grumbled through a frown. The "new" you begins each day posed in front of the bathroom mirror and grinning your way through 15 seconds of Ha-Ha-Hee-Hee-Ho-Hos from The Laughter Prescription. You will feel the joy as you fill and refill this Happiness Rx from your own INNER pharmacy.

Yes, you have a cellular pharmacy that can be accessed 24 hours a day, and all you need to get a refill is to learn how to ACT on the combinations that unlock, open and disperse your happy medicine.

Expect quizzical looks as you make this role transformation. "Is that really you?" they may ask. Or, "What's the *real* reason you're

---

"How old would you be if you didn't know how old you was?"
SATCHEL PAIGE

acting so happy?" "Did you win the lottery, or what?" Grin back and tell them, "I'm finally getting my ACT together." Yes, laughter is contagious and hopefully, in time, you will have your entire family and friends laughing, not at you, but WITH you.

To get into this new role, you must rehearse. Great actors don't just waltz on stage and give performances worthy of standing ovations the first time they speak their lines. No, they spend hours and hours practicing their lines and their moves over and over again until they get the timing, the inflection of the voice and the body movement all in sync. At the dress rehearsal and on opening night, they keep practicing to improve their part. Each and every "staging" is an opportunity to perfect the part. Just as actors do, physicians practice, too. As do we all in every role we choose to play or wish to conquer. Practice doesn't make perfect but it surely improves subsequent performances.

AGEless Wisdom

Get better smileage out of life.

Actors put themselves in the roles of thieves, jokers, ailing patients, whining children, heroes, sheroes and many others. They manufacture the chemistry (feelings) that allows them to be that character.

And, when you act the UPbeat happy part, you can reap other dividends. Not only health but social and financial gains. For instance, phone marketers, by looking into a mirror and smiling as they make their calls, will sell 17 percent more because a smile is not only seen, but heard. And waiters and waitresses who put on the "happy act" will make 27 percent more tips. After all, if a customer picks up on your laughter and smiles, they will feel it and they are inclined to come back or buy more. You can bank on IT!

But acting the happy part offers personal perks, too. You automatically gain better posture and project a fun-loving attractiveness that draws others to you like a magnet. Have you ever been *pulled* into a group because of laughter? Of course you have.

And why? Because you feel better joining that group. The wisdom of Mother Nature tells you so. What are feelings again? Of course, they're chemistry. And happy chemistry makes us joyfully WELLderly.

In other words, you become healthier, happier, and more successful by consciously modeling or acting like or associating with happy, laughing people—even if you have to FAKE it at first.

Get Physical

You need to rehearse your body as well as your mind. So, let's get physical! The most healing power of all is the magic of movement. Getting regular exercise is probably the single best thing we can do for our bodies. The best news is that you're never TOO OLD to start exercising!

Women and men aged 60 to 75 who were previously sedentary but got involved in supervised walking or stretching/toning programs started to feel good about themselves. That's the finding from a recent study published in the *Annals of Behavioral Medicine*. The study tracked older adults who began exercising three times a week for six months. The participants walked at indoor malls or strength-trained with resistance bands. They reported feeling WELL about their physical condition, appearance and strength.

Here are SEVEN Oscar-winning reasons to tone UP with exercise:

SEVEN Oscar-winning reasons to tone UP with excercise:

1. You can s-l-o-w down your aging process.
2. You can reduce stress.
3. You can dodge many joint and back pains.
4. You can bolster your overall flexibility and muscle strength.
5. You perk up your posture and fortify your bones.
6. You enhance your immune system to protect you against infections.
7. You gain added protection from heart disease, diabetes, stroke and other chronic conditions.

See! There are MANY benefits of healing with motion. And, to get into your "new" role, you can do so with little to no sweat—honest! And even have more fun! Now here's an added bonus: You will APPLAUD the happy role you build UP.

Back UP!

As mentioned in ACT 4, for you folks needing a little extra help to obtain more youthful posture, I've got just the "tools" you need. Years of poor posture will result in tight, inelastic tissue. You need to loosen UP this tissue before you can attain—and maintain—good posture.

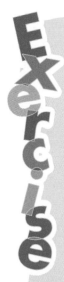

Let's start by warming up those low back muscles. Shed the stiffness with this 60-second back-arching exercise:

- Lie on your stomach on the floor and get into a "push-up" position by placing your hands palm down in front of your shoulders.

- Push up, keeping your entire body from your hips down pressed firmly on the floor. Focus on arching your lower back. Then gently lower yourself to the floor.

- Do 10 of these arch-up stretches. Try to hold each of the last arches for a count of 10.

Also, do some upper back (not neck) arch exercises by using a rolled up sheet or by arching over the back of a firm, padded chair with the arms raised over your head.

A few words of caution: please stop doing these stretching exercises if you start to feel dizzy or if the stretching causes pain (a little hurting is often a good sign that means your back needed a good stretching). Please get your physician's approval before doing these exercises if you are over age 60 or have a chronic health problem. Do not perform these exercises if you have been diagnosed with spinal stenosis, scoliosis, or spondylolisthesis.

If it's a pain to laugh, my best-selling book, *Muscle Pain Relief in 90 Seconds,* may help reduce or eliminate some nagging or chronic muscle pains. The FOLD and HOLD Method examined in this book (in its 8th printing and in four languages) clarifies the self-mobilizing "right moves" used by Mother Nature to erase common, nagging muscular aches and pains. And we all know that Mother knows best! The book explains how aches and pains go away over night (never during the day), when one sleeps like a baby. It identifies comfortable positioning of the body that will help unlock many common muscular problems such as headaches, neck aches, backaches, tennis elbow, golfer's elbow, carpal tunnel syndrome, plantar fasciitis, hip pain, and more. This simple, easy-to-learn technique relieves many muscular pains so that you can turn UP the capacity to laugh.

Now Stomach This

Okay! You've got your pains relieved and your back muscles warmed up. Time to tone up your stomach muscles. Here are two quick exercises you can perform anywhere, anytime—even while chatting on the phone, standing in line, or doing a sink full of dishes. The beauty of these exercises is that the movements can be so subtle that folks around you may not even realize you're "working out."

#1: Suck in your abdominal muscles and hold them firmly for five to 10 seconds. Expect a little "hurt" when you are tightening them. Do this repeatedly. In the car, on the phone, watching television.

#2: Imagine that you're a belly dancer—without the costume and castanets and the pelvic grind. Just use the (suck it in, let it out) belly moves. Tighten your stomach muscles inward and then let them out to a musical beat.

My patient, Sam Torkelson, said "Sometimes I do this exercise in front of the mirror while doing the Laughter Rx (see ACT 4) or listening to music. After a shower, when the fogged-up mirror hides the bare facts of reality, I can imagine being a Medicare Chippen-DALE." Now there is some positive "scripting" and not a "pretty sight." But it got Sam's laughter going and endorphins generated. As it did mine.

And did you know that when you strive to sit tall and stand tall, you can actually lose weight! Sitting and standing up straight requires more energy than sitting slouched. At any age, practicing proper sitting posture can burn 10 to 15 calories per hour. In a year (don't worry, I already did the math for you), that could equate to losing 10 to 15 pounds of fat!

And, when you stand and get ready to move, try walking with a bounce to your step instead of a shuffle. A stage posturing practice called the Alexander Technique suggests imaging a thread lifting up from the top of the head so that you are standing up straight and essentially being lifted with every step. It's a light, soft step walk. In a way, the Alexander Technique is much like the first half of that famous Muhammad Ali quote: "Float like a butterfly..." You'll find that your round shoulders will become magically upright and you will feel less anxious. Because that spring in your step is generating a chemistry message to your muscles to "lighten UP." Try it!

Remember "The Liquidation Diet" from ACT 3. By combining the sit and stand postures and watching what you drink, WAIST-FULL fat will just melt away!

Exercise Any Time, Any Where

Regular balancing exercise, especially for VPs (Vintage People) is important to help prevent falls and broken bones. Here are a couple no-sweat steps to "rehearse" every day: Walk heel-to-toe for 10 to 20 steps on level ground so that your heel is just in front of the toes of the opposite foot each time you take a step. You can also stand on one foot for 15 to 20 seconds anywhere, even while waiting in the supermarket line.

You can take these tips a "step" further. Researchers at the Mayo Clinic in Rochester, Minnesota (where I trained to become a board-certified surgeon) report that older folks who practice tai chi (a gentle, slow-moving form of ancient Chinese martial arts) reduced

> ## AGEless Wisdom
> Laughter is inner jogging.
> NORMAN COUSINS

their risk of falling by 40 percent and improve their balance. This martial art also promotes relaxation and builds stamina. So, sign up for a tai chi class in your community—or, at least rent a tai chi video from your local library and become "WELL balanced."

Or, you could become a "splash" hit. The Arthritis Foundation recommends that older women with arthritis loosen up and do endurance exercises to strengthen their hearts and make their lungs more efficient so that they can fight fatigue. The Arthritis Foundation also recommends that the WELLderly should (with their doctors' approval) consider swimming or doing water aerobics in chest-high or shallow water for 20 to 30 minutes a few times a week. The buoyancy of water helps support their bodies and keeps stress off their spine, hips, knees, and feet. Select a heated pool—especially if you're like me and live in a *c-o-l-d* place like Minnesota. Water temperature should be between 83 and 90 degrees.

Conduct Yourself WELL!

Here's something you did as a child. So tune in once again to your youthful HIGH notes. Now it's time to re-learn how to "conduct" yourself WELL. Tap into that fantastic orchestra within and learn how to **J**og with the **ARM**s. I call it **J'ARM**. Professional musical conductors are **J'ARM**ers. They experience and enjoy the benefits of **J**ogging with their **ARM**s to music. Great symphony orchestra conductors live, on average, FIVE years longer than average. And they are healthier in both mind and body than others their age.

You can learn more about "**J'ARM**ing," from my book, *The Orchestra Conductor's Secret To Happiness and Long Life.*

But don't take my word for it. In 1980, the Metropolitan Life Insurance Company published its findings of a longevity study of conductors. In examining 437 active and former conductors, researchers reported that mortality among conductors was 38 percent BELOW their contemporaries in the general population.

Here are a few conductors who really loaded up the candles on their birthday cakes:

Leopold Stokowski – 95
Arthur Fiedler – 85
Bruno Walter – 86

Even Leonard Bernstein, who died at the relatively young age of 72, lived a long life despite his many "vices." "God knows, I should be dead by now," Bernstein said a couple years before his death. "I smoke. I drink. I stay up all night. I'm over committed on all fronts. I was told that if I didn't stop, I'd be dead at 35. Well, I beat the rap."

Musical conductors truly enjoy making those grand, sweeping motions of their arms while engulfed in a sea of sound.

There is a bit of a conductor inside each of us. We just need to re-tap and turn UP our childhood memories and ACTions. Many of us would prance and dance around our parents' living room pretending to lead a marching band or a large orchestra. We would hoist our arms high in the air and march around to the music. Or better yet, dance with the arms, legs and whole body flowing as the waves of joyful music surrounded us. And sometimes there were alone times in front of the mirror leading "imaginary friends" and admiring our own performance.

J'ARMing gives you the excuse to be childlike again, to let yourself go with the musical flow and reinvigorate both your mind and body. You're encouraged to grab a baton (imagined or real) and recapture that excitement, that feeling of being in control, of moving out of yourself, of leaving stress and pain in their tracks. Indeed, J'ARMing provides more fun than you can "shake a stick at!"

J'ARMing requires no pricey equipment or special wardrobe. It is not hindered by Mother Nature's weather wrath and there's no jolting impact to your hip, knees, or feet.

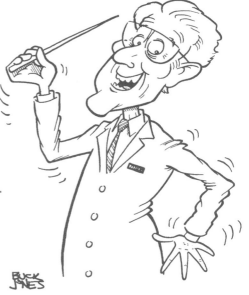

As Doctor Seuss might say,

You can **J'ARM** in the park.
You can **J'ARM** in the dark.
You can **J'ARM** as a lark.

You can **J'ARM** in a chair.
You can **J'ARM** on a stair.
You can **J'ARM** in the BARE.

You can **J'ARM** here,
there,
You can **J'ARM**
ANYWHERE!

In fact, moving your arms, or even imagining waving your arms in the air to a favorite song, can offer 12 positive benefits:

Twelve positive benefits to waving your arms in the air:

1. Improved posture
2. Bolster muscle strength and flexibility
3. Improved circulation
4. Better balance
5. Weight loss
6. A gentle shoulder and back massage
7. Reduction of your physiological and mental ages
8. A positive attitude and readiness for laughter
9. A "wash" for your brain that removes annoying distractions and makes you smarter
10. Higher self-esteem
11. Elevation of endorphins and other feel-good brain chemicals
12. For stroke patients, it may help reconnect some of the injured neural pathways

Before you start waving your baton (which can be a ballpoint pen, spoon, silk scarf, tongue depressor, back brush from the shower or even a peacock feather), I offer two suggestions:

#1 – Let go a little. Bring out the childlike qualities and approach this more as play than exercise.

#2 – Select UPbeat music. Even more ideally, choose a song with UPlifting lyrics so that the positive message can help raise your "inner uppers"—the endorphins. Pick a piece of music that strikes a personal chord and raises the spirits.

Here is a personal WELLderly **J'ARM** favorite. It has been around a long time. You may have lived IT UP and sung IT OUT with friends as a kid. Now, let's bring it back and "stick with it." If performed with a group—you will "stick together"—and have more fun than "you can shake a stick at."

SMILE

(To the tune of Battle Hymn of the Republic)

It isn't any trouble just to s-m-i-l-e,
It isn't any trouble just to s-m-i-l-e,
So smile when you're in trouble;
It will vanish like a bubble,
If you only take the trouble just to s-m-i-l-e.

It isn't any trouble just to l-a-u-g-h,
It isn't any trouble just to l-a-u-g-h,
So laugh when you're in trouble;
It will vanish like a bubble,
If you only take the trouble to l-a-u-g-h.

It isn't any trouble just to g-r-i-n, grin
It isn't any trouble just to g-r-i-n, grin
So grin when you're in trouble;
It will vanish like a bubble,
If you only take the trouble just to g-r-i-n, grin

Ha-ha, Ha-ha Ha-ha Ha-ha Ha-ha Ha-ha Ha
Ha-ha, Ha-ha Ha-ha Ha-ha Ha-ha Ha-ha Ha
Ha-ha Ha-ha Ha-ha Ha;
Ha-ha Ha-ha Ha-ha Ha,
Ha-ha Ha-ha Ha-ha Ha-ha Ha-ha Ha-ha Ha

Okay TUNE UP, grab the baton, turn ON the music, and even better, stand in front of a full-length mirror to see your entire "performance." If you're worried that your neighbors may think that you're a little nuts, draw the blinds OR, better yet—invite them to face the music and join you! Live IT UP, together!

When you are ready, conduct yourself WELL! Raise your arms up high. Move your arms comfortably in all directions as a conductor does to the music's beat. Have some fun and do so with painless exaggeration and with enthusiasm. If unable or if painful, just imagine the movements. There's no right or wrong. Sing along with the music—who cares if you're a little off-key? Remind yourself that you are the conductor. Allow yourself to feel the music. If you wish, increase your aerobic benefits by standing or dancing or marching around.

And take sneak peeks at yourself in the mirror. Take a mental "snapshot" of the grinning STAR and conjure up and reIN-ACT that happy image throughout your day. Over and over and over again.

Kudos! You've become a J'ARMing Lady or a Prince J'ARMing! BRAVO!

Ageless Ally

As Helen Gray unloads her golf bags from the trunk of her car, you can't help but notice the button pinned to her vest. It reads: "Born to putt."

Meet Helen, an 83-year-old retired nurse from Tustin, California. She answered the patriotic call to duty during World War II and enlisted as a Navy nurse assigned to the South Pacific. After the war, she spent 40 years as a hospital nurse and a caring mother of three.

The day she retired from nursing in 1962 was the day she chose to start the sport of golf. She has more than made up for lost time on the links, often winning her women's golf league's putt contests.

Envious golfers three and four decades younger than her respectfully call her "One-putt Helen."

It may take Helen several fairway strokes to reach the green, but once she does, she rarely two-putts the ball into the hole. On the 18-hole course, Helen's best putting performance was 25 putts!

Do the math and you'll discover that equates to 1.3 putts per hole. Most golfers feel happy when they take only two putts on a hole, which would total a very respectable 36 putts for the game.

And, she accomplishes this while pulling her cart up and down the hills and walking the entire course.

"Many golfers just want to chip onto the green and then on the next stroke, aim for the hole," says Helen. "Not me. Whenever I near the green, I always take dead-aim for the flagstick. I'm always thinking about sinking the ball into the hole, not just getting close."

Her golfing philosophy offers us a bigger lesson on how to approach life. Why be tentative, why just go for the comfortable choice when you can set your sights on your true goals, ambitions?

Why, indeed.

Helen Gray

ACT

YOU MADE "IT"!
The Show Goes On!

Congratulations! You are becoming a star by learning to IN-act the happy, healthy part with conviction. You are earning rave notices from all the reviewers—including yourself. With diligent practice and preparation, you have earned center stage billing after learning to IN-act a better, and in many ways, a new happier, healthier role with realism and conviction. You feel great. You look great. BRAVO!

Now, you're anxious to direct and help others to get their acts together, too. But CAN you usher others—including your friends, neighbors, and families—into new acts? Inevitably, after delivering a lecture or seminar, several from the audience approach me. "Dr. Anderson, I have this friend who is always in such a tragic part." Or, "What can I do to make my husband or my wife or my fellow worker feel happier?"

The answer is always the same: you CAN'T change another person's act. You can't simply hand them a "new HAPPY script" to read and expect them to slip into this new role. You are unable to turn ON and turn UP their feel-good chemistry. You can't wave a magic

"If I were given the opportunity to present a gift to the next generation, it would be the ability for the individual to learn to laugh at himself."
CHARLES SCHULZ

wand and—*poof!*—make them happier and healthier. Or even make them want to become happier and healthier.

Alas, your unhappy friends and family must do their role chang-ing for and by themselves. And it does not occur overnight. That said, however, you can certainly cast your influence over them by acting as their happy and healthy role models. You can project a

> **AGEless Wisdom**
>
> It's not how old you are that counts, but how you are old.

living example of how to turn ON and become REAL in an UPbeat role. And they more than likely, by association, will eventually catch your infectious ACT. It is contagious.

In essence, you can become their HE-ro or SHE-ro. You become the person who exemplifies the power of TRANCE-forming, TRANCE-acting and TRANCE-mitting this powerful physiological message. You show them how by doing IT. Subliminally, you help them raise the curtain on their future happiness.

Since ancient Greek days, every performer has a role model whom they emulate. Today, method actors watch and rehearse, watch and rehearse, and then watch and rehearse AGAIN how their talented idols do IT. The students emulate these role models through personal association or by watching their stage, movie or television performances for a complete head-to-toe and inside-the-soul character study. Eventually, a TRANCE-formation occurs as the student IN-acts the new chemistry.

People who perform on the stage know they must INNERtain before they can entertain. They must BE there before they ARE there. They must become INstilled with and catch UP with the appropriate INNER chemistry before they can put on a winning performance. Before they can pass their chemistry across life's footlights, before they can turn ON the desired feelings of the audience. Only when an actor performs his or her part WELL and with REAL feelings will the audience catch this INNER chemistry, too. And only then, will the audience "get IT."

Great actors know when they've got IT. And it's only when they've got IT that they can pass IT on. The performer must have IT and IT must be REAL before the audience can GET IT. *In Never Act Your Age,* we spotlight the chemistry of the happy, healthy, successful part. Only after a person has that part IN-acted as a staged habit will IT become REAL.

All your life you have known people who have IT. Where do they get that spark, composure, presence and that aura that emits energy and attracts others? What is IT? You've already discovered in this book that feelings are chemistry and chemistry is feeling. The feeling that is IT is the feeling of beneficial, healthy chemistry—those extraordinary endorphins and other positive neuropeptides. Hence, the on-target expression: *By Jove, you've got IT!*

Use your IT to become a HIT. The best way to have an "unhappy person" convert to happiness is to have them "catch IT" from a person who is already infected with the happy chemistry. Spreading this HAPPY-demic sure beats spreading the common cold—*achoo!* Or worse, anger and hate.

> **AGEless Wisdom**
>
> We don't stop playing because we're old: we grow old because we stop playing.

As a VP (Vintage Person), perhaps one of our greatest missions in life is to be that "classic" player who helps "direct" our society, our family (especially our grandchildren) onto the stage of happiness, health and success.

Grandchildren—Our Ultimate Understudies

Do Chinese-speaking kids come from Chinese-speaking families? Do Italian-gesturing kids spring from Italian-gesturing families? Do kids acquire the beliefs, the talk, the walk of their elder role models? Do the emotions of grandparents spread to our grandchildren?

Of course, the answer to all four questions is a resounding YES.

Consequently, the young, our children and grandchildren, are our ultimate understudies. It is our goal, our desire that someday they will take center stage with the knowledge, tools and skills to play a happy part WELL. They will have the inner chemistry to make this a better world. A society that will feel more comfortable and inviting. With our help, they will make all of this happen. They will realize how to design, apply and play their happy parts WELL, to make this a dramatically better world.

Regretfully, we have all seen many of our peers—Vintage Persons

AGEless Wisdom
He/she who laughs, lasts.

(VPs) who have not been exemplary role models. Too often, we have seen people who are out of shape, tense, grumpy, achy and/or fatigued much of their waking hours. Many who are abusive to themselves and consequently to others. We don't want their bad habits to "steal the scene" and influence our grandchildren. Regrettably, these miserable actors will have some affect on our grandchildren. But the WELLderly STARS like you will have a much greater impact on them. Because fun people and fun times are remembered and re-LIVED.

We can't predict or mandate what will happen in our world. We can only hope to leave a living legacy to future generations. We can leave them with positive memories, images, examples, and role models that they can emulate. A role that they can IN-act and pass on, again and again to future generations.

As a VP, the principal legacy I can leave to my grandchildren—Britta, Ethan, Beckett, and Elise—is to constantly practice and portray a happy, fun, UPbeat, WELLderly character who has his part so well IN-acted that they and their children will become beneficiaries of my passion for life.

Realize that:

> **"Children Are
> Living MESSAGES
> We Send to a Time
> We Will Not See."**

Yes, children are our legacy, our charge, and our destiny. As WELLderly role models we can help future generations make this a better world. By youth witnessing UPbeat characters to emulate they will masterfully develop their own role WELL. Sunrise, Sunset, so go the days, the years. And they too will pass from youth, to middle age, and ultimately to a starring WELLderly role of their own.

So, the next time you spend time with your grandchild, please remember:

"No written word or mortal plea can teach young hearts what they should be. Nor all the books upon the shelves but what the teachers are themselves."

Rally Your Friends and Family

Staying connected to a large supporting cast and fostering a large number of behind-the-scene stagehands is essential to IN-acting the WELLderly role. The best way to reap the benefits of friendly, happy connections is to teach the UPbeat ACT—by example. Become the INstructor who plants the seeds of happiness WELL and then harvests a joyful bumper crop of future INNERtainers.

As the WELLderly, we can connect with family as friends. It's important enough to repeat! That which connects us more than anything else is to play out and to teach our happy part. Yes, teach IT and teach IT well. We teach IT by example and by everything we do because the understudies are always off-stage, watching. They may appear or pretend not to be observing our every ACT-ion, but they are watching every move, every voice inflection. They will someday become a part of us—and we will always be a part of them.

Sports teams often speak of the "home field advantage." What is this home field advantage? After all, the fans or cheerleaders aren't the ones who are scoring touchdowns or making three-point baskets. The players are. Yet, when cheered UP by a roaring, applauding, supporting crowd and a sideline of rah-rah cheerleaders, the home team can rally to claim amazing come-from-behind victories. How does this happen? This "home field advantage" is feel-good chemistry. The fans have IT and the players get IT and IT is a winner.

You don't need a sports arena to cash in on this home field advantage. This game of life "chemistry" can also be experienced in our clubs, in our places of worship, in our businesses, our neighborhoods, and where we live. As the WELLderly, you are encouraged to serve as coaches and cheerleaders for others. My patients are told, "I can't play the game (of life) for YOU, but I will coach and cheer you ON. I will revel if you score, but win or lose, there will be fun in 'playing the game.'"

To take on your ultimate role—that of a coach, or director, you need to see how you "reflect" on both yourself and on others. If you are fired UP and are a respected role model, you will be a success at any part you choose to play. After all, folks don't want to go to a sick doctor. You don't want to visit a doctor who smokes or one who is extremely overweight. Nor do you want to receive exercise tips from a fitness instructor who is always munching on jelly donuts and always having to buy larger sizes of sweatpants. You won't return to a salesperson who doesn't smile. And—one can't learn to be happy from a person who is sad, grumpy or angry.

The point? To become a happier, healthier, WELLderly person one needs to choose the right role models for health and success.

The easy choice for the WELLderly is to remain or become *child-like* (not childish) and laugh for the sheer "health of it."
Never to Act Your Age!

And the Best Connector Is... a Smile

Connecting. In theater, actors who play UP the happy part must connect with their audiences. It is this invisible tether that keeps audiences entertained and sometimes on the edge of their seats or rolling in the aisle from full-belly laughter. In society, we can also connect through sharing smiles, expressing pleasantries, practicing random acts of kindness and the ultimate: volunteerism.

Out of that terrible 9/11 tragedy, we learned that the USA is indeed the UNITED States of America. People started smiling more at strangers on the street, talking, sharing and helping. Becoming volunteers. It is the spirit (chemistry) of the street, of the city, of the nation that has been IN-hanced—not diminished—since that fateful day.

Hopefully, through "Dr. Dale's Laughter Prescription," the J'ARMing and other helpful METHOD acting advice in this book, you will be recognized as a WELLderly Age Sage who conducts yourself WELL. As the happy Age Sage, you will convey the mood, the feeling, the chemistry that there will always be a better day ahead; that there will always be another opening, another show. In this present moment, why not be happy? We've got nothing to lose.

AGEless Wisdom

Grin and Share IT!

Of course, realistically, we know that eventually our earthly run will come to a close. Eventually, we will be playing a more heavenly role. But until then, we must strive to live it UP right here—right through the last encore. And, when the final earthly curtain falls, an appreciative audience will applaud you for "an act WELL done!"

But until that time, the show must go on! And ON! And ON! We have a hit and it is becoming better the longer it plays. The message of this book is about going on with the show, not about the final curtain call. *Never Act Your Age* is about getting and keeping the ACT together. About the excitement of staging and re-staging a new fun show. A performance, full of joy, love and laughter that you IN-ACT WELL.

Light the lights.
Curtain UP!
You're ON!
ACT NOW and
Keep Laughing for "THE HEALTH OF IT."
MORE! ENCORE! ENCORE!
You've got no place to hit but the HEIGHTS!

BRAVO!

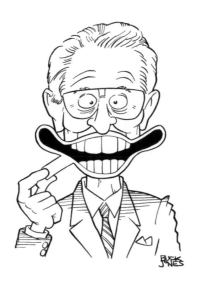

Ageless Ally

Larry Wilson

Powerful. Dynamic. Wise. These three words aptly describe Larry Wilson.

And, add FUN.

Wilson, a best-selling author, speaker, and management consultant, has created five successful companies. At 71, this father of 6 and grandfather of 11 happily admits that he is still growing up.

"Growing old is a necessity, but growing up is a choice," says Wilson, of Wayzata, Minnesota. "I don't feel old, think old, or wake up wondering how long I'll live. I tell people to take a bigger bite out of life and live it fully."

Wilson's road to emotional and financial success has been a bumpy ride. He grew up with a short-tempered alcoholic father. He married three times. He lost a child to leukemia.

"All these represent imprints on my life," says Wilson, author of *Play to Win! Choosing Growth Over Fear* (Bard Press). "These experiences helped me later in life. I learned a lot of coping skills, that everything may not be wonderful and sweet, but how you can turn some of life's emotional scars into competencies."

Wilson addresses corporate audiences and often speaks of winning. But his definition of victory is one that empowers all.

"Winning, to me, is all about giving your very best and how you respond to life," he says. "Winning is not about competition. Too often, people in business and in life play not to lose. They rely on a survival strategy rather than a growth strategy. True winners embrace spontaneity, learn from life's curveballs, and live their lives not to prove themselves, but to express themselves."

And, Wilson says, he stays young by finding time to listen to music and by never turning down a chance to play tennis.

"People who say that they don't have time to play, hear, or share music are overdeveloped survivors and underdeveloped achievers," he says. "Tennis, like music, also represents a metaphor for life. It offers great exercise, fun, companionship, and gives you the chance to focus and stay in the present."

APPENDICES

**The Paraphrased, Massaged and Doctored Wisdom
of Constantin Stanislavski**

ACTitude Assessment

Crib Sheet

Play It UP!!!

More UP Words

Dr. Dale's Laughter Prescriptions

Resources/References

Other Books by Dale L. Anderson, M.D.

The Paraphrased, Massaged and Doctored Wisdom of Constantin Stanislavski (1863-1938)

- The METHOD OF ACTING was not invented. It was founded on the physical and spiritual laws governing the nature of humanity!

- The METHOD OF ACTING is a creative process of living and experiencing organically a desired role. This METHOD OF ACTING enables YOU to create the image of that desired role—breathe the life of human spirit into that character and then—by natural means—embody it with artistic beauty.

- YOU must be the master of your own INSPIRATION (chemistry) and know how to call it forth at the hour announced. This is the secret of the art of becoming a successful WELLderly person.

- To play the WELLderly role, YOU must know how to put on and wear a costume, and how to use proper body language and stage props appropriately. YOU can do this only when you feel YOURSELF in the part and the part in YOURSELF.

- Bring YOURSELF to the point of IN-ACTing a new role concretely. AS IF it were YOUR life. And when YOU sense this real kinship, then this newly created being will become soul of YOUR soul and flesh of YOUR flesh. This AS IF acting is a lever to lift YOU into a world of a new chemistry.

- YOU, the WELLderly, must above all believe in what is happening around YOU and in what YOU are doing. Truth cannot be separated from belief, nor belief from truth. YOU must believe in what YOU say and do and YOU will be convincing.

- For YOU to establish the right WELLderly state it is essential to work step by step to establish HABITS. Piecemeal this habit system enters YOU until IT (the chemistry) becomes incorporated as second nature. At all times and in all places the WELLderly person must constantly practice to achieve a true (chemistry) feeling.

- This capacity to transform YOURSELF, body and soul, is the prime requirement for a successful WELLderly performance. Acting a WELLderly part is a whole way of life. YOU cannot do it all at once.

- YOU develop a talent to be WELLderly. And the more talent YOU develop the more YOU will care about technique.

- Then for YOU, the WELLderly,
  the difficult becomes habitual,
  the habitual becomes easy
  and the easy becomes BEAUTIFUL!

From Constantin Stanislavski's books (1) *An Actor's Handbook* (2) *An Actor Prepares* and (3) *Building a Character.* Paraphrased, "massaged and doctored" by Dale L. Anderson, M.D., www.acthappy.com. ("WELLderly" = "actor.")

ACTitude Assessment

Getting My Act Together

Achieve—and maintain—a happy, healthy (and wealthy) mind-body connection with this ACT-itude assessment guide. Here's a partial list of activities and thoughts that make you FEEL good, pick you UP and turn you ON. Ask yourself:

- What are my aromas of fun-funny/happy/healthy?
- What are my colors of fun-funny/happy/healthy?
- What are my tastes of fun-funny/happy/healthy?
- What are my sounds of fun-funny/happy/healthy?
- What are my costumes of fun-funny/happy/healthy?
- What are my postures/poses of fun-funny/happy/healthy?
- What are my movements of fun-funny/happy/healthy?
- What are my props of fun-funny/happy/healthy?
- Who are my supporting players of fun-funny/happy/healthy?
- Who are my role models of fun-funny/happy/healthy?
- What makes me laugh out loud—at work, home, alone?
- What is my happiest/funniest TV show, book, cartoon, joke, movie, pun?

You can BANK on them. Curtain UP! You're ON! ACT NOW!

© Copyright: Dale L. Anderson, M.D., J'ARM, Inc., 2982 West Owasso Blvd., St. Paul, MN 55113 • email: DrDLA@acthappy.com • www.acthappy.com

Crib Sheet—FUN, Happy, Healthy ACT UP, OUT and FORWARD

Body:

Expand, broaden, widen, arch, stretch, reach, roll, open, push, move UP, OUT, FORWARD. Focus on your head, neck, shoulders, back, arms, legs, and hands. Supple and light.

Face:

Eyebrows arched up, forehead up, mouth and lips in a smile. Keep the face mobile, changing, radiant, and alert.

Eyes:

Open wide, sparkling, shining, flashing, searching, seeing and making contact.

Thoughts:

Be "a part of" not "apart from," think in terms of "you, we and us," happy, positive, sensual, searching, exploring, developing, and out-going.

Motion:

Stable, strong, sure steps, bouncing and dancing.

Breath:

Steady, deep, strong inhalations that expand the chest UP, OUT, FORWARD followed by strong, steady or explosive exhalations.

Voice:

Louder, higher, faster, varied musical tone/rhythm/tempo/pitch.

Hygiene:

Hair, skin, teeth, nails and clothes clean and styled.

Condition:

Balance, stability, strength, flexibility, energy.

Skin:

Warm, moist, smooth, soft, clean.

Colors/Costume:

Bright, light, flashy, varied, patterned—fashionable.

Taste/Aroma:

Pleasing, fresh, natural—chocolate, peppermint, cinnamon, popcorn—your favorite.

Stage:

Arranged, charted, planned, uncluttered, safe and clean.

Cast:

Familiar, friendly, supporting, welcoming, attractive, cheerful.

Rehearse:

Studied, prepared, readied.

Play It UP!!!

Here's my all-star cast of favorite UP words:

Body: UP, stand UP, sit UP, straighten UP, stretch UP, open UP, pump UP, puff UP—with head UP, arms UP, palms UP, thumbs UP, and measure UP.

Face: UP, chin UP, cheeks UP, mouth UP, laugh it UP.

Eyes: UP, lids UP, look UP, spark UP, light UP.

Think: UP, psych UP, wire UP, bring UP, dream UP, study UP, book UP, life UP, "what's UP," play it UP.

Move: UP, come UP, rise UP, jump UP, spring UP, step UP, lighten UP, bounce UP, pep UP, push UP, reach UP, stay UP, hold UP.

Breath: Fill UP, laugh it UP, shout out (up), burst out (up), laugh out loud.

Voice: Speak UP, drum UP, tune UP, turn UP, listen UP, ring UP, call UP.

Costume: UP, dress UP, suit UP, touch UP, make UP, spruce UP, doll UP, get UP, color UP.

Hygiene/groom: Clean UP, fix UP, wash UP, shine UP, do UP, brush UP, make UP, touch UP.

Condition: UP, shape UP, work UP, strengthen UP, tone UP, bone UP, buff UP.

Touch: UP, warm UP, heat UP, fire UP, feel UP to it.

Taste: Dish UP, spice UP, eat UP.

Stage: Rig UP, set UP, build UP, fix UP.

Cast: Pair UP, team UP, meet UP, mix UP, marry UP.

Rehearse: Study UP, practice UP, and you'll be UP to it.

MORE UP WORDS

Laugh UP the ENDORPHINS with INNER UPPER words and get "HIGH" ON LIFE!!

If you are up to "righting UP" some uplifting word plays
here is a longer list of "kid-friendly" UP words
(See page 63 for sharing creative "Right UPs")

Act Up	Clean UP	Fill UP
Add UP	Come UP with ___	Finish UP
Back UP	Come UPpance	Fired UP
Bear UP	Cook UP	Fix UP
Beat UP	Cover UP	Follow UP
Blow UP	Crack UP	Fork UP
Board UP	Cut UP	Game's UP
Boil UP	Dig UP	Gang UP
Bone UP	Dish UP	Gas UP
Book UP	Do UP	Get UP
Bottle UP	Dolled UP	Give UP
Bottoms UP	Double UP	Go UP in smoke
Break UP	Draw UP	Goof UP
Bring UP	Dredge UP	Grow UP
Brush UP	Dress UP	Gum UP
Buck UP	Drink UP	Had it UP to ____
Bust UP	Drum UP	Ham it UP
Butter UP	Ease UP	Hand UP
Call UP	Eat UP	Hang UP
Catch UP	End UP	Heads UP
Check UP	Eyes UP	Healed UP
Cheer UP	Face UP to it	Heat UP
Chin UP	Feeling UP to it	High UP
Choke UP	Fed UP	Hit UP
Choose UP	Figure UP	Hold UP
Clam UP	First UP	Hung UP

Hunt UP

Hurry UP

Hush UP

Jack UP

Jig is UP

Jump UP

Keep UP

Keyed UP

Laid UP

Lap it UP

Laugh it UP

Let Up

Lift UP

Light UP

Line UP

Listen UP

Lit UP

Live it UP

Look UP to

Looking UP

Loosen Up

Make UP

Mark UP

Married UP

Measure UP

Meet UP

Mend UP

Mix UP

Mop UP

Move UP

Muscle UP

Once UPon a time

Open UP

Order UP

Own UP

Pack UP

Pair UP

Palms UP

Pass UP

Patch UP

Pay UP

Pep UP

Perk UP

Pick UP

Pile UP

Pin UP

Pipe UP

Play UP to

Play it UP

Psyched UP

Pop UP

Puffed UP

Pull UP

Pump UP

Push UP

Put UP (a front)

Rack UP

Rig UP

Ring UP

Rise UP

Roll UP

Round UP

Rub UP

Run UP

Runner UP

Rustle UP

Save UP

Scrape UP

Send UP

Set UP

Settle UP

Seven UP

Shape UP

Shine UP

Shoot UP (grow)

Show UP

Sidle UP

Sign UP

Sit UP

Size UP

Slip UP

Slow UP

Snap UP

Soften UP

Sow UP

Speak UP

Speed UP

Spice UP

Split UP

Spring UP

Spruce UP

Square UP

Stack UP

Stand UP (for)

Start UP

Stay UP

Steamed UP

Step UP

Stick UP

Stir UP

Stock UP

Stop UP

Store UP	Turn UP	UP day
Strike UP	Wait UP	UP for grabs
Stuffed UP	Wake UP	UP for the ____
Sum UP	Walk UP	UP front
Swallow UP	Warm UP	UP in arms
Swell UP	Wash UP	UP in the air
Tack UP	What's UP	UP on luck
Take UP	Whip UP	UP person
Talk UP	Whoop it UP	UP to date
Team UP	Wind UP	UP to Heaven
Tear UP	Wired UP	UP to it
Think UP	Wise UP	UP to one's ____
Thumbs UP	Work UP	UP to par
Tie UP		UP to scratch
Time's UP	UP a creek	UP to something
Tone UP	Up a sleeve	UP to the minute
Toss UP	Up a street	UP, UP and away
Touch UP	UP a tree	UPper hand
Track UP	UP and at 'em	UPpers
Trump UP	UP and coming	UPs and downs
Tune UP	UP and UP	UPsadaisy

Drawn UP by Dale Anderson, M.D.

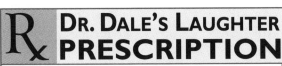

R_x DR. DALE'S LAUGHTER **PRESCRIPTION**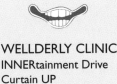

NAME:

ADDRESS:

WELLDERLY CLINIC
INNERtainment Drive
Curtain UP
America
www.ActHappy.com

In front of mirror

Belly Laugh

15 seconds, 2x/Day

R_x DR. DALE'S LAUGHTER **PRESCRIPTION**

NAME:

ADDRESS:

WELLDERLY CLINIC
INNERtainment Drive
Curtain UP
America
www.ActHappy.com

In front of mirror

Belly Laugh

15 seconds, 2x/Day

RESOURCES/REFERENCES

Joel Goodman, founder of The Humor Project, Inc. and author of *Laffirmations: 1001 Ways to Add Humor to Your Life and Work* (Health Communications, Inc., 1995). Web site: www.humorproject.com

Madan Kataria, M.D., founder of Laughter Club International, and author of *Laugh for No Reason*. Web site: www.indiabuzz.com/laughter/

Allen Klein, author of *The Healing Power of Humor and The Courage to Laugh*. Web site:www/allenklein.com

Steve Wilson, co-founder of the World Laughter Tour. Author of *Eat Dessert First*. Web site: www.worldlaughtertour.com

Patty Wooten, R.N., registered nurse and therapeutic humorist. Web site: www.jesthealth.com

Association of Applied Therapeutic Humor, Web site: www.aath.org

American Holistic Medical Association, Web site: www.holisticmedicine.org

Recommended Books

Herbert Benson, M.D. *Timeless Healing: The Power and Biology of Belief*

Bill Cosby *Time Flies*

Norman Cousins *Anatomy of an Illness* and *Head First: The Biology of Hope*

Deepak Chopra, M.D. *Ageless Body, Timeless Mind: The Quantum Alternative to Growing Old*

Viktor Frankl *Man's Search for Meaning*

Maryann Glasgow with Dale Anderson, M.D. *Gift to the Present: Wellderly Wisdom*

Dean Ornish, M.D. *Program for Reversing Heart Disease: The Only System Scientifically Proven to Reverse Heart Disease without Drugs or Surgery.*
Robert Ornstein, Ph.D. and David Sobel, M.D. *Healthy Pleasures: Discover the Proven Medical Benefits of Pleasure and Live a Longer, Healthier Life.*
Michael F. Roizen, M.D. *Real Age: Are You as Young as You Can Be?*
Martin Seligman *Learned Optimism*
David Snowdon, Ph.D. *Aging with Grace: What the Nun Study Teaches Us About Leading Longer, Healthier, and More Meaningful Lives.*
Larry Wilson *Play to Win: Choosing Growth Over Fear in Work and Life.*

Other Books By Dale L. Anderson, M.D.

The Orchestra Conductor's Secret to Health and Long Life, John Wiley and Sons, Inc., 1997, $11.95.

Act Now!, Chronimed Publishing, 1995, $11.95

Muscle Pain Relief in 90 Seconds: The Fold and Hold Method, John Wiley and Sons, Inc., 1995, $12.95. (8th printing, four languages).

Gift to the Present: Wellderly Wisdom by Maryann Glasgow with Dale Anderson, M.D., Beaver's Pond Press, Inc., 2002, $14.95

To schedule Dr. Anderson to speak for upcoming events or to order his books and other and HAPPY-demic products, please refer to his web site: www.acthappy.com.

RESOURCES/REFERENCES

Joel Goodman, founder of The Humor Project, Inc. and author of *Laffirmations: 1001 Ways to Add Humor to Your Life and Work* (Health Communications, Inc., 1995). Web site: www.humorproject.com

Madan Kataria, M.D., founder of Laughter Club International, and author of *Laugh for No Reason*. Web site: www.indiabuzz.com/laughter/

Allen Klein, author of *The Healing Power of Humor and The Courage to Laugh*. Web site:www/allenklein.com

Steve Wilson, co-founder of the World Laughter Tour. Author of *Eat Dessert First*. Web site: www.worldlaughtertour.com

Patty Wooten, R.N., registered nurse and therapeutic humorist. Web site: www.jesthealth.com

Association of Applied Therapeutic Humor, Web site: www.aath.org

American Holistic Medical Association, Web site: www.holisticmedicine.org

Recommended Books

Herbert Benson, M.D. *Timeless Healing: The Power and Biology of Belief*

Bill Cosby *Time Flies*

Norman Cousins *Anatomy of an Illness* and *Head First: the Biology of Hope*

Deepak Chopra, M.D. *Ageless Body, Timeless Mind: The Quantum Alternative to Growing Old*

Viktor Frankl *Man's Search for Meaning*

Maryann Glasgow with Dale Anderson, M.D. *Gift to the Present: Wellderly Wisdom*

Order Form

Order Form

Order these books by Dale Anderson, M.D.

	QUANTITY	AMOUNT	TOTAL
Never Act Your Age	_____	$14.95	_____
The Orchestra Conductor's Secret to Health and Long Life	_____	$11.95	_____
Act Now!	_____	$11.95	_____
Muscle Pain Relief in 90 seconds: the Fold and Hold Method	_____	$12.95	_____
Gift to the Present Wellderly Wisdom by Maryann Glasgow	_____	$14.95	_____
Tax: MN Residents add 6.5%			_____
Subtotal			_____
Shipping Charges	1st book	$ 4.00	_____
for each additional book		$ 1.00	_____
TOTAL			_____

❏ Please send information about Dr. Anderson's Speaking Programs

Please send check or money order to:
Dale L. Anderson, M.D.
2982 West Owasso Blvd
St. Paul MN 55113

Ship to:

Name _____

Address_____

City _____ State _____ Zip _____

credit card orders accepted online at: acthappy.com
or toll free 1-800-901-3480